Blastic Plasmacytoid Dendritic Cell Neoplasm

Editor

ANDREW A. LANE

HEMATOLOGY/ONCOLOGY CLINICS OF NORTH AMERICA

www.hemonc.theclinics.com

Consulting Editor
GEORGE P. CANELLOS
EDWARD J. BENZ, Jr

June 2020 • Volume 34 • Number 3

ELSEVIER

1600 John F. Kennedy Boulevard • Suite 1800 • Philadelphia, Pennsylvania, 19103-2899

http://www.theclinics.com

HEMATOLOGY/ONCOLOGY CLINICS OF NORTH AMERICA Volume 34, Number 3
June 2020 ISSN 0889-8588, ISBN 13: 978-0-323-72260-5

Editor: Stacy Eastman
Developmental Editor: Kristen Helm

Hematology/Oncology Clinics (ISSN 0889-8588) is published bimonthly by Elsevier Inc., 360 Park Avenue South, New York, NY 10010-1710. Months of issue are February, April, June, August, October, and December. Business and Editorial Offices: 1600 John F. Kennedy Blvd., Ste. 1800, Philadelphia, PA 19103—2899. Customer Service Office: 3251 Riverport Lane, Maryland Heights, MO 63043. Periodicals postage paid at New York, NY and at additional mailing offices. Subscription prices are $443.00 per year (domestic individuals), $876.00 per year (domestic institutions), $100.00 per year (domestic students/residents), $480.00 per year (Canadian individuals), $100.00 per year (Canadian students/residents), $1085.00 per year (Canadian institutions) $547.00 per year (international individuals), $1085.00 per year (international institutions), and $255.00 per year (international students/residents). International air speed delivery is included in all *Clinics* subscription prices. All prices are subject to change without notice. **POSTMASTER:** Send address changes to *Hematology/Oncology Clinics of North America*, Elsevier Health Sciences Division, Subscription Customer Service, 3251 Riverport Lane, Maryland Heights, MO 63043. Customer Service (orders, claims, online, change of address): Elsevier Health Sciences Division, Subscription **Customer Service, 3251 Riverport Lane, Maryland Heights, MO 63043. Tel: 1-800-654-2452 (U.S. and Canada); 314-447-8871 (outside U.S. and Canada). Fax: 314-447-8029. E-mail: journalscustomerservice-usa@elsevier.com (for print support); journalsonlinesupport-usa@elsevier.com (for online support).**

Reprints. For copies of 100 or more, of articles in this publication, please contact the Commercial Reprints Department, Elsevier Inc., 360 Park Avenue South, New York, New York 10010-1710; Tel.: 212-633-3874, Fax: 212-633-3820, E-mail: reprints@elsevier.com.

Hematology/Oncology Clinics of North America is covered in *MEDLINE/PubMed (Index Medicus), EMBASE/ Excerpta Medica, and BIOSIS.*

Contributors

CONSULTING EDITORS

GEORGE P. CANELLOS, MD
William Rosenberg Professor of Medicine, Department of Medical Oncology, Dana-Farber Cancer Institute, Boston, Massachusetts, USA

EDWARD J. BENZ Jr, MD
Professor, Pediatrics, Richard and Susan Smith Professor, Medicine, Professor, Genetics, Harvard Medical School, President and CEO Emeritus, Office of the President, Dana-Farber Cancer Institute, Boston, Massachusetts, USA

EDITOR

ANDREW A. LANE, MD, PhD
Director, BPDCN Center, Division of Hematologic Neoplasia, Division of Adult Leukemia, Department of Medical Oncology, Dana-Farber Cancer Institute, Harvard Medical School, Boston, Massachusetts, USA

AUTHORS

L. ELIZABETH BUDDE, MD, PhD
Assistant Professor, Department of Hematology and Hematology Cell Transplantation, City of Hope, T Cell Therapeutics Research Laboratory, Irell & Manella Graduate School of Biological Sciences, Beckman Research Institute, City of Hope, Duarte, California, USA

MOHAMAD CHERRY, MD
Morristown Medical Center, Atlantic Hematology Oncology, Morristown, New Jersey, USA

ERIC DECONINCK, MD, PhD
Professor, Hematology, Service Hématologie, Université de Bourgogne Franche-Comté, INSERM Unite Mixte de Recherche (UMR) 1098, RIGHT Interactions Greffon-Hôte-Tumeur/Ingénierie Cellulaire et Génique, Centre Hospitalier Universitaire de Besançon, Besancon Cedex, France

FRANCINE GARNACHE OTTOU, PhD
Université de Bourgogne Franche-Comté, INSERM Unite Mixte de Recherche (UMR) 1098, RIGHT Interactions Greffon-Hôte-Tumeur/Ingénierie Cellulaire et Génique, Etablissement Français du sang Bourgogne Franche Comté, Besançon, France

MONICA L. GUZMAN, PhD
Associate Professor, Division of Hematology and Medical Oncology, Weill Cornell Medical College, New York, New York, USA

MICHAEL HADDADIN, MD
Research Scholar, Department of Medicine, Memorial Sloan Kettering Cancer Center, New York, New York, USA

DANIELLE HAMMOND, MD
Fellow, Department of Leukemia, The University of Texas MD Anderson Cancer Center, Houston, Texas, USA

JESSE P. HIRNER, MD
Department of Dermatology, The Center for Cutaneous Oncology, Dana-Farber Cancer Institute, Brigham and Women's Hospital, Harvard Medical School, Boston, Massachusetts, USA

MOHAMED A. KHARFAN-DABAJA, MD, MBA, FACP
Division of Hematology-Oncology, Blood and Marrow Transplantation Program, Mayo Clinic, Jacksonville, Florida, USA

ANDREW A. LANE, MD, PhD
Director, BPDCN Center, Division of Hematologic Neoplasia, Division of Adult Leukemia, Department of Medical Oncology, Dana-Farber Cancer Institute, Harvard Medical School, Boston, Massachusetts, USA

NICOLE R. LEBOEUF, MD, MPH
Department of Dermatology, The Center for Cutaneous Oncology, Dana-Farber Cancer Institute, Brigham and Women's Hospital, Assistant Professor, Harvard Medical School, Boston, Massachusetts, USA

YIXIAN LI, MD
Pediatric Hematology, Oncology, Marrow and Blood Cell Transplantation, Children's Hospital at Montefiore, Bronx, New York, USA

JOHN T. O'MALLEY, MD, PhD
Department of Dermatology, The Center for Cutaneous Oncology, Dana-Farber Cancer Institute, Brigham and Women's Hospital, Assistant Professor, Harvard Medical School, Boston, Massachusetts, USA

ANNA PAWLOWSKA, MD
Pediatric Hematology, Oncology and Hematopoietic Stem Cell Transplantation, City of Hope, Duarte, California, USA

NAVEEN PEMMARAJU, MD
Associate Professor, Department of Leukemia, The University of Texas MD Anderson Cancer Center, Houston, Texas, USA

TONY PETRELLA, MD
Department of Pathology, University of Montréal, Hôpital Maisonneuve-Rosemont, Montréal, Quebec, Canada

STEFANO PILERI, MD, PhD
Division of Diagnostic Haematopathology, European Institute of Oncology, IRCCS, Milan, Italy

KANA SAKAMOTO, MD, PhD
Researcher, Pathology Project for Molecular Targets, Researcher, Division of Pathology, The Cancer Institute, Japanese Foundation for Cancer Research, Tokyo, Japan

MARIA ROSARIA SAPIENZA, MS, PhD
Division of Diagnostic Haematopathology, European Institute of Oncology, IRCCS, Milan, Italy

MAYUMI SUGITA, MD
Research Associate, Division of Hematology and Medical Oncology, Weill Cornell Medical College, New York, New York, USA

VICTORIA SUN, PhD
Pediatric Hematology, Oncology and Hematopoietic Stem Cell Transplantation, City of Hope, Duarte, California, USA

WEILI SUN, MD, PhD
Pediatric Hematology, Oncology and Hematopoietic Stem Cell Transplantation, City of Hope, Duarte, California, USA; Janssen Pharmaceuticals, Los Angeles, California, USA

KENGO TAKEUCHI, MD, PhD
Project Leader, Pathology Project for Molecular Targets, Chief, Division of Pathology, The Cancer Institute, Japanese Foundation for Cancer Research, Center Chief, Clinical Pathology Center, The Cancer Institute Hospital, Japanese Foundation for Cancer Research, Tokyo, Japan

JUSTIN TAYLOR, MD
Assistant Member, Department of Medicine, Leukemia Service, Memorial Sloan Kettering Cancer Center, New York, New York, USA

TONGYUAN XUE, MD
Graduate Student, Departments of Hematology and Hematology Cell Transplantation, and Molecular Medicine, T Cell Therapeutics Research Laboratory, Irell & Manella Graduate School of Biological Sciences, Beckman Research Institute, City of Hope, Duarte, California, USA

Contents

Clinical and biological presentation of patients with blastic plasmacytoid dendritic cell neoplasm (BPDCN) is depicted to highlight criteria that might alert physicians. Diagnosis of BPDCN is still challenging and requires (1) immunophenotyping of blood or bone marrow aspiration using several markers (CD4, CD56, HLA-DR, myeloid and lymphoid lineage markers) and should include pDC markers such as CD123, cTCL1, CD303, and CD304, and/or (2) pathologic analysis of cutaneous lesions, also with immunohistochemistry using markers specific to BPDCN.

Blastic plasmacytoid dendritic cell neoplasm (BPDCN) is a rare, aggressive malignancy derived from the plasmacytoid dendritic cell that commonly involves the skin. Cutaneous involvement is often the initial presentation, with deep purple or red-brown macules, plaques, or tumors. As such, dermatologists may be the first to see these patients and, in addition to oncologists, should be familiar with its presentation to facilitate early diagnosis, helping to distinguish it from acute myelogenous leukemia cutis.

Blastic plasmacytoid dendritic cell neoplasm (BPDCN) is a rare hematologic neoplasm with a dismal prognosis and no standard therapy. In the past, its cellular ontogenesis was obscure, and BPDCN had been erroneously named CD56$^+$/TdT$^+$ blastic NK cell tumor and CD4$^+$/CD56$^+$ hematodermic neoplasm. Finally, in 2008, the BPDCN was correctly recognized as a neoplasm deriving from the malignant transformation of plasmacytoid dendritic cell precursors and classified among the myeloid neoplasms. Since then, the understanding of BPDCN biology has improved rapidly: the DNA mutational status of BPDCN has been extensively investigated revealing a spectrum perfectly resembling its myeloid lineage derivation.

Blastic plasmacytoid dendritic cell neoplasm (BPDCN) is a skin-tropic hematopoietic malignancy. Approximately 60% of cases with analyzable

Blastic plasmacytoid dendritic cell neoplasm (BPDCN) is a rare, difficult-to-diagnose, highly aggressive myeloid malignancy with poor prognosis and no standard of care. The interleukin-3 receptor α, or CD123, is highly expressed in patients with myeloid malignancies, particularly acute myeloid leukemia and BPDCN. CD123 is overexpressed on leukemic stem cells compared with normal hematopoietic stem cells, suggesting CD123 as an attractive immunotherapeutic target. To date, multiple CD123-targeted therapeutic avenues have been explored to treat BPDCN and other CD123$^+$ hematologic malignancies. This review summarizes immunotherapies targeting CD123 for the treatment of BPDCN and related neoplasms.

Blastic plasmacytoid dendritic cell neoplasm (BPDCN) is an orphan hematologic malignancy with poor outcomes. Tagraxofusp (SL-401) was the first drug approved specifically for patients with BPDCN, in 2018. Additional therapeutic strategies are still needed to improve survival and minimize treatment-related toxicity. This article outlines novel targeted approaches that are in preclinical or clinical development for BPDCN. Although there is no known targetable genetic abnormality that defines BPDCN, data from functional testing of primary tumors, gene expression analyses, and adaptation of targeted drug approaches from other cancers to BPDCNs harboring specific mutations have nominated several promising strategies.

Blastic plasmacytoid dendritic cell neoplasm (BPDCN) is a rare, aggressive hematological malignancy, derived from plasmacytoid dendritic cells. It mainly occurs in older adults, but has been reported across all age groups. Most patients present with skin lesions with or without marrow involvement and leukemic dissemination. Treatment with high-risk acute lymphoblastic leukemia therapy regimens with central nervous system prophylaxis is recommended in pediatric patients. Stem cell transplant in children is recommended for relapsed/refractory disease or high-risk disease at presentation. New targeted therapies including the recently FDA-approved anti-CD123 cytotoxin show great promise in improving the response rate.

Blastic plasmacytoid dendritic cell neoplasm (BPDCN) has to be considered an orphan tumoral disease. BPDCN is a good model concerning the structuring and the organization of a concerted medical program on a nation-based, transnational, or international level. In 2019 in France the diagnosis process for BPDCN was clearly established. Two prospective clinical trials are ongoing. Because of the difficulties in diagnostic procedures and the rarity of the disease it is important that European countries collaborate to build a real European network to ensure the best and equitable medical care to all BPDCN patients.

Mohamed A. Kharfan-Dabaja and Mohamad Cherry

Blastic plasmacytoid dendritic cell neoplasm (BPDCN) is a rare aggressive hematologic malignancy derived from precursors of plasmacytoid dendritic cells. Historically, BPDCN has had few available treatment options and a poor prognosis. The emergence of novel targeted therapies, namely tagraxofusp, has changed the treatment landscape of BPDCN, but data are lacking regarding the long-term durability of responses. Despite absence of randomized data, allogeneic hematopoietic cell transplant has become the de facto option for patients with BPDCN who achieve a first complete remission. As new therapies continue to emerge, it will be important to evaluate the role of postallograft maintenance/consolidation.

HEMATOLOGY/ONCOLOGY CLINICS OF NORTH AMERICA

SERIES OF RELATED INTEREST

Surgical Oncology Clinics of North America
https://www.surgonc.theclinics.com/

THE CLINICS ARE AVAILABLE ONLINE!
Access your subscription at:
www.theclinics.com

HEMATOLOGY/ONCOLOGY CLINICS OF NORTH AMERICA

FORTHCOMING ISSUES

August 2020
Follicular Lymphoma
Jonathan W. Friedberg, Editor

October 2020
Mantle Cell Lymphoma
John P. Leonard, Editor

December 2020
Systemic Amyloidosis due to Monoclonal Immunoglobulins
Raymond L. Comenzo, Editor

RECENT ISSUES

April 2020
Myelodysplastic Syndromes
David P. Steensma, Editor

February 2020
Contemporary Topics in Radiation Medicine, Part II: Disease Sites
Ravi A. Chandra, Lisa A. Kachnic, and Charles R. Thomas, Jr, Editor

December 2019
Contemporary Topics in Radiation Medicine, Part I: Current Issues and Techniques
Ravi A. Chandra, Lisa A. Kachnic, and Charles R. Thomas, Jr, Editors

SERIES OF RELATED INTEREST

Surgical Oncology Clinics of North America
http://www.surgonc.theclinics.com/

THE CLINICS ARE AVAILABLE ONLINE!

Access your subscription at:
www.theclinics.com

Preface

Blastic Plasmacytoid Dendritic Cell Neoplasm in 2020 and Beyond

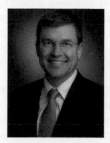

Andrew A. Lane, MD, PhD
Editor

Blastic plasmacytoid dendritic cell neoplasm (BPDCN) is an aggressive blood cancer with poor patient outcomes. Relatively little was known about the pathobiology and therapeutic sensitivities of the disease until recently. Consequently, the approach to the patient was uninformed, empiric, and inadequate.

However, much has changed in the last decade, and the outlook for patients with BPDCN is improving. Disease classification and differential diagnosis have been formally codified. Awareness among hematologists, oncologists, pathologists, and dermatologists (BPDCN, while closely related to acute myeloid leukemia [AML], manifests with skin lesions in most patients) is increasing. Laboratory studies have concentrated on understanding BPDCN genetics, mechanisms of dendritic cell transformation, and unique therapeutic vulnerabilities. BPDCN-focused prospective clinical trials are being performed worldwide, most often in the setting of newly formed multicenter cooperative groups given the relative rarity of patients with the disease in any single institution.

These initial efforts have produced some answers to the question, what is BPDCN? In 2020, we have a better understanding of how BPDCN is related to other hematologic malignancies and the ways it is unique. Laboratory work has nominated several new therapeutic targets of interest in BPDCN, some of which are shared with other blood cancers. The greatest clinical research success to date was a multicenter phase 2 registration trial that led to the first Food and Drug Administration approval of a treatment specifically for BPDCN, tagraxofusp-erzs (also known as SL-401 or DT-IL3). This recombinant fusion protein consisting of interleukin-3 fused to a truncated diphtheria toxin payload is also the first-in-class molecule targeting CD123, the alpha subunit of the interleukin 3 receptor. CD123 is highly expressed in BPDCN tumor cells, but also in several other hematologic malignancies, including AML, where it is a marker

Hematol Oncol Clin N Am 34 (2020) xiii–xiv
https://doi.org/10.1016/j.hoc.2020.02.011
0889-8588/20/© 2020 Published by Elsevier Inc.

hemonc.theclinics.com

of leukemia stem cells. Thus, lessons learned from targeting CD123 in BPDCN may be important across other blood cancers.

In this issue, we present a set of articles that cover the state-of-the-art understanding and management of BPDCN in 2020. We cover BPDCN clinical presentation, diagnosis, and disease pathology, including molecular/genetic features and CD123 as a critical marker and therapeutic target. Clinical management is discussed, including conventional chemotherapy and tagraxofusp. Novel emerging treatments for BPDCN in various stages of preclinical and clinical research are covered, including small molecules, immunotherapies, and rational combination approaches with tagraxofusp, chemotherapy, and other agents. We also present articles on unique aspects of BPDCN in children, and the approach to the disease in Europe, where targeted therapies are not yet available. Finally, we close with data on stem cell transplantation in BPDCN.

There have been major leaps in understanding and treating BPDCN since it was officially named in 2008. Patients are benefiting from disease-specific research and a community of academic "BPDCN-ologists" who have worked together to move the field forward. The stage is set for many new discoveries in the future that will be directly relevant to further improving outcomes in this previously orphan disease.

Andrew A. Lane, MD, PhD
BPDCN Center
Division of Hematologic Neoplasia
Division of Adult Leukemia
Department of Medical Oncology
Dana-Farber Cancer Institute
Harvard Medical School
450 Brookline Avenue, Mayer 413
Boston, MA 02215, USA

E-mail address:
Andrew_Lane@dfci.harvard.edu

Blastic Plasmacytoid Dendritic Cell Neoplasm
Clinical Presentation and Diagnosis

Eric Deconinck, MD PhD[a], Tony Petrella, MD[b],
Francine Garnache Ottou, PhD[c],*

KEYWORDS

- BPDCN • Diagnosis • Morphologies • Immunophenotyping • Anatomopathology
- Clinical presentation

KEY POINTS

- Patients with blastic plasmacytoid dendritic cell neoplasm (BPDCN) are typically older men who first exhibit colored cutaneous lesions that precede dissemination by a few months.
- Typical morphologies of blastic cells include medium size, cytoplasm with irregular basophilia, and small vacuoles under the cytoplasmic membrane and large pseudopodia in a fraction of the population.
- Diagnosis requires phenotypical or immunochemistry confirmation of the pDC origin using specific markers.

The clinical presentation of blastic plasmacytoid dendritic cell neoplasm (BPDCN) can be heterogenous, although a typical profile has emerged.[1–3] The patient with BPDCN is typically an older man who first exhibits one or several persistent cutaneous lesions leading to various examinations. Subsequently, some weeks or months later, he develops progressive pancytopenia with specific complications (anemia, bleeding, and infectious complications), as is the case in overt acute leukemia presentations. Sometimes there also may be tumoral visceral involvement.[1,4–11]

[a] Service Hématologie, Université de Bourgogne Franche-Comté, INSERM Unite Mixte de Recherche (UMR) 1098, RIGHT Interactions Greffon-Hôte-Tumeur/Ingénierie Cellulaire et Génique, Centre Hospitalier Universitaire de Besançon, 3 Boulevard Alexandre Fleming, Besançon Cedex 25030, France; [b] Department of Pathology, University of Montréal, Hôpital Maisonneuve-Rosemont, 2900 Boulevard Edouard-Montpetit, Montréal QC H3T 1J4, Quebec, Canada; [c] Université de Bourgogne Franche-Comté, INSERM Unite Mixte de Recherche (UMR) 1098, RIGHT Interactions Greffon-Hôte-Tumeur/Ingénierie Cellulaire et Génique, Etablissement Français du sang Bourgogne Franche-Comté, 8 rue du Dr JFX Girod, Besançon 25000, France
* Corresponding author. 8, rue du Docteur Jean-François-Xavier Girod, BP1937, Besançon Cedex 25020, France.
E-mail address: francine.garnache@efs.sante.fr

Hematol Oncol Clin N Am 34 (2020) 491–500
https://doi.org/10.1016/j.hoc.2020.01.010
hemonc.theclinics.com
0889-8588/20/Crown Copyright © 2020 Published by Elsevier Inc. All rights reserved.

Multiple case reports or retrospective series of adult patients have shown a median age of 60 (53–68) years and a male-to-female ratio of 3 or 4 to 1.[12–18] It should also be noted that pediatric cases exist, and although rare, have been clearly documented.[19] Recent publications reported a possible bimodal distribution, with a first peak of incidence in patients younger than 20 years, and a second peak after the age of 60.[6,12] In a recent large series,[5] we confirmed a median age of 64 (11–89) years and a predominance of 4 men for 1 woman. We also identified older age and altered general status as adverse clinical prognostic features with a significant impact on overall survival. The adverse impact of age is present as a continuous variable, that is, the older the patient, the worse the prognosis. General status is also important, but is significantly altered in only 10% to 15% of patients.[5]

Cutaneous lesions are the hallmark of the disease and are present in more than 90% (60%–100%) of patients reported in the literature.[20–26] Skin lesions can be of various size (millimeters to centimeters), color (red, purple, xanthochromic), and forms (solitary or multiple nodules, plaques). They are usually nonpruritic and present as a bruiselike infiltration with no preferential anatomic localization, except a trend to involve the upper thoracic integument. With time, these lesions can progress to a scaly presentation. The skin is the first step of the disease in 60% to 90% of the cases.[18,21,24,26,27] In our experience, cutaneous involvement is present in 85% of patients and precedes marrow infiltration by 2 to 3 months in 45% of cases.[5] A single cutaneous lesion was present in 46.5%, whereas disseminated skin involvement was visible in 38%, and the disease remained localized to the skin in only 1.5% of patients. The presence of isolated lesions is a marker of better clinical outcome, whereas an eruptive presentation is probably the sign of aggressive disease, with reported progression-free survival of 23 versus 9 months, respectively.[26] The skin could be considered as a sanctuary organ for BPDCN tumoral cells and probably a significant reflection of the tumor burden of disease.[10,18,26] Real BPDCN cases without any skin disease have been reported, exhibiting no other specific clinical trends, and this does not confer a different prognostic course on them.[1–3,28] On the contrary, cases with tumoral involvement limited to the skin with no further spread of the disease in the blood, marrow, or other organs have also been described, but they remain rare, and exhibit a potentially better prognosis.[6,21,27,29] In clinical trials, the evaluation of skin involvement should be based on the experience of dermatologists with the quantification of the tumoral mass of the skin using a specific tool, that is, the severity-weighted assessment tool, which will enable valuable comparisons between different series.[8,30,31]

Tumoral mucosal involvement has been described in very few cases, preferentially affecting the oral cavity and mimicking fungal infections or nasal NK-T lymphoma presentation.[32–34]

The marrow is the second most frequently affected organ in patients with BPDCN, explaining why many patients are initially suspected of overt acute leukemia with complications related to cytopenia and cutaneous lesions.[1,5,10,15]

Other visceral involvements concern the lymph nodes, which can be affected in approximately half of patients, with no preferred anatomic area.[1,5,9–11,13,15] The spleen and liver also can be affected in up to 20% of cases. No specific tropism for the gastrointestinal tract has been described. All organs can be affected, although reports remain anecdotal (breast, lung, bladder, or kidney for instance).[5,27] They are clinically perceptible, rarely compressive or asymptomatic, and individualized only after computed tomography scan or metabolic exploration.[10,18]

A major clinical point is the neurologic involvement at initial diagnosis. In some series, up to 30% of central nervous system (CNS) involvement is described.[1,8,23,35,36] This consists of the presence of tumoral cells in the cerebrospinal fluid without any neurologic signs, or rarely, in a classic meningeal syndrome or some localized neurologic deficit. In our recent series, clinical neurologic involvement was documented in 8% of cases with 2 cases of symptomatic ocular infiltration.[5]

Because of the diversity of clinical presentation, oncologists, hematologists, internal medicine physicians, and dermatologists must all be aware of this specific tumoral entity, to avoid misleading diagnosis and ensure adequate and rapid medical care of the patient.

DIAGNOSIS OF BLASTIC PLASMACYTOID DENDRITIC CELL NEOPLASM IN CLINICAL PRACTICE
Morphology

Leukemic pDC blastic cells frequently and rapidly disseminate in the blood and bone marrow, leading to a leukemic presentation with which physicians and biologists are confronted. These professionals should therefore be aware of the presentation of BPDCN in the hematology laboratory, based on morphologies of the blastic population and the immunophenotypic profile that can be observed.

Cytopenia is frequent at diagnosis in relation to bone marrow involvement; anemia and thrombocytopenia in two-thirds of patients, and less frequently, neutropenia.[1,5,11] Biologists can suspect BPDCN based on the morphologic characteristics of the blastic population on blood or bone marrow aspiration smears. Most frequently, blasts are intermediate-sized cells with a round, frequently peripheral nucleus, with open chromatin and frequent nucleolus. Cytoplasm displays faint basophilia with irregular gray areas and no granulation. Frequently, but only in a fraction of the blastic population, cells show very small or coalescent vacuoles under the cytoplasmic membrane and large pseudopodia (**Fig. 1**). Importantly, biologists must be aware that morphologies can be different and challenging. Difficulties arise in cases with small pseudo-lymphoid cells, with less blastoid chromatin, mimicking lymphoma; large, strongly basophilic cytoplasm leading to pseudo-monoblastic cells, mimicking monoblastic leukemia; or undifferentiated cells with no or very infrequent cells with vacuoles and pseudopodia. An immunoblastoid cytomorphology was also described in 2018,[37–43] associated with MYC rearrangements and a CD56-immunophenotype, with a prevalence of approximately 35% in Japanese populations, and which seems to be lower in Caucasians (4%–8%).[7,44–47]

It is noteworthy that the frequency of cases with circulating blasts or bone marrow involvement at diagnosis is variable, depending on the origin of the published series. It is frequent (±70% of cases) when the diagnosis is made by hematologists,[1,5,11,48,49] but lower when the diagnosis is made by dermatologists due to investigation of one or more first skin lesions.[32] This is not surprising, because isolated cutaneous lesions seem to precede leukemic diffusion in most cases.

In 10% to 20% of cases, BPDCN arises in patients known to have myelodysplastic syndrome or in patients presenting dysplasia on myeloid cells,[50,51] suggesting that the development of BPDCN represents a second event in a context of myelodysplasia.[50,52,53]

High incidence of CNS involvement[1,16,51,54] implies that cerebral liquid could be evaluated in search of blastic cells by cytology analysis or flow cytometry, both at diagnosis and at suspected relapse, where it is even more frequent, and probably underestimated (30% to almost 100% of cases).[1,54]

Immunophenotype

Identifying BPDCN is not difficult when the CD45^{low} blastic population lacks all myelomonocytic, erythroid, megakaryocytic, lymphoid, and plasma cell lineage markers.

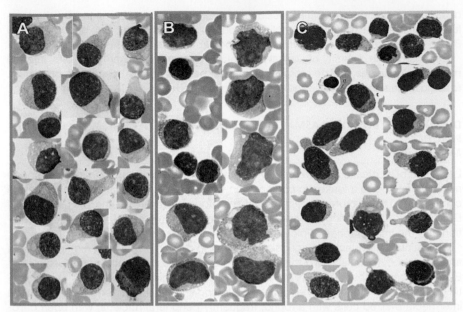

Fig. 1. Typical morphologies of BPDCN cells in blood or bone marrow aspirates. (*A–C*) Three cases are shown. The blastic population is intermediate-size cells with a nucleus that is frequently eccentrically located and a gray, lightly basophile coloration of the cytoplasm with some clearer areas. Only a fraction of the population presents large pseudopodia and microvacuoles like a rosary under the cytoplasmic membrane. Some cells present larger vacuoles. May-Grunwald-Giemsa stain, original magnification ×1000. (*Courtesy of* Francine Garnache-Ottou, Besançon, France.)

Only CD4 and CD56 are expressed with a high level of HLA-DR. However, this phenotype is not specific to BPDCN, because monoblastic leukemia, for example, can harbor these markers. The pDC lineage origin must be confirmed by the evaluation of (more or less) pDC-specific marker expression, such as CD123 (interleukin-3-R alpha), CD303 (BDCA2), and cTCL1 (T-cell leukemia 1).[55–57] CD123 is not specific to BPDCN because B-cell (B-ALL) and T-cell acute lymphoblastic leukemia (T-ALL) and more frequently acute myeloid leukemia (AML) also can express it.[22,58–60] However, the level of CD123 expression is statistically higher in BPDCN,[61] thereby giving a first indication to suggest this diagnosis, if this type of blastic population is identified with very high CD123 expression (the level is at least as high as that of basophils). CD304 is also frequently expressed in BPDCN, but is not specific to the pDC lineage, because it can be expressed by B-ALL[62] and monoblastic cells.[61] CD303 is very specific, but not very sensitive, because nearly 30% of BPDCNs lose this marker, or its expression is very low by flow cytometry, and interpretation is difficult.[61] cTCL1 is a proto-oncogene expressed during B-cell and T-cell development, and that is absent on mature T-cell and myeloid lineages. It is overexpressed in mature lymphoid malignancies[63] as well as in B-ALL and some AMLs,[55] but it is expressed at higher levels in BPDCN.[55]

As BPDCN frequently expresses myeloid or lymphoid lineage markers (eg, CD7, CD33, CD117, or CD22)[64,65] and even some markers that are very specific to lymphoid lineage, such as cCD79a[51] and cCD3,[4] the diagnosis of BPDCN may not be immediately evident. Moreover, BPDCN can harbor low CD56 expression or may lack CD56[10,23,66,67] and more rarely, lack CD4.[68] It is clear that diagnosis is still challenging, and confirming the pDC origin using a wide range of markers, such as CD123, CD303, CD304, and cTCL1, is mandatory to achieve BPDCN diagnosis by flow cytometry.

BPDCN must be differentiated to mature pDC proliferations associated with myeloid neoplasm (MPDCP)[22,69–71] described in the World Health Organization 2017 classification,[4,72] which associates aggregates of pDCs that are always CD56⁻ and a myeloid malignancy, such as chronic myelomonocytic leukemia most often, or myelodysplasia or AML.[73] In MPDCP associated with AML, an excess of CD56⁻ pDC is associated with a CD34⁺ blastic population.[4,74] BPDCN in a large majority of cases lacks immature markers, such as CD34 and CD133 (except for TdT, which is expressed in one-third of cases).[46] It has been suggested that MPDCP cases could be considered as immature BPDCN,[23] but this remains to be explored.

Pathology

The diagnosis of BPDCN might require a biopsy specimen, particularly for patients without a leukemic phase. As most of the patients are presenting a skin involvement, the diagnosis is regularly made by skin biopsy. Sometimes the diagnosis is made on lymph node or bone marrow biopsies.

Skin biopsy generally shows a dense and monomorphous infiltrate involving dermis and fat tissue. The epidermis is generally spared with presence of a grenz-zone. The infiltrate is constituted of medium-sized cells that display a slightly irregular-shaped nucleus with smooth chromatin resembling lymphoblasts. One or several medium or small-sized nucleoli can be seen. The cytoplasm is difficult to visualize and never exhibits granulation. Large and small-sized cells can be seen within the infiltrate of medium-sized cells but are generally rare. Inflammatory infiltrate also may be present but most often is slight and mainly consists of small T lymphocytes. Commonly, there are no plasma cells or eosinophils within the infiltrate. Mitoses are seen in variable number. Angiocentrism and angiodestruction are uncommon features. Cutaneous appendages are generally erased by the tumor cell infiltration. When involved, the lymph nodes are generally, at least initially, infiltrated with a leukemia pattern, involving the interfollicular areas and medulla first, sparing B-follicles. In patients with a leukemic phase, the bone marrow is generally infiltrated. The bone marrow biopsy may show either a mild interstitial or diffuse infiltrate. Furthermore, the hematopoietic tissue may exhibit dysplastic features, especially dysplastic megakaryocytes and may show an increased number of monocytes.

Immunohistochemistry is mandatory to achieve the final diagnosis. As discussed above, a panel of antibodies is required including CD123, CD4, CD56, TCL1, CD3 and CD20. Typical BPDCN shows CD123, CD4, CD56 and TCL1 positivity and CD3 and CD20 negativity.

SUMMARY

Overall, biologists and pathologists need to be alert to the diagnosis of BPDCN, and they should learn to recognize its characteristics. Because it is rare and depends on recognition, physicians are confronted with this diagnosis much less frequently than with acute leukemia or cutaneous lymphoma. Diagnosis can be made on blood or bone marrow aspiration, if infiltrated, using a large panel of antibodies including BPDCN markers, or on pathologic analysis of cutaneous lesions, also with immunohistochemistry using markers that enable clear differentiation of BPDCN from immature or myeloid leukemia and also MPDCP.

ACKNOWLEDGMENT

The authors would like to thank Fiona Ecarnot, the *Groupe Français d'hématologie cellulaire* (GFHC), the *Groupe d'etude immunologique des leucémies* (GEIL) and the *Société Française d'hématologie* (SFH). This study was supported by INCA (PRT-K-15-175), PHRC (PHRC-K16-93), the ligue contre le cancer (CCIRGE - BFC), the association Cent pour sang la vie and by the association "Laurette Fugain".

DISCLOSURE

The authors have nothing to disclose.

REFERENCES

1. Pagano L, Valentini CG, Pulsoni A, et al. Blastic plasmacytoid dendritic cell neoplasm with leukemic presentation: an Italian multicenter study. Haematologica 2013;98:239–46.
2. Rauh MJ, Rahman F, Good D, et al. Blastic plasmacytoid dendritic cell neoplasm with leukemic presentation, lacking cutaneous involvement: case series and literature review. Leuk Res 2012;36:81–6.
3. Wang H, Cao J, Hong X. Blastic plasmacytoid dendritic cell neoplasm without cutaneous lesion at presentation: case report and literature review. Acta Haematol 2012;127:124–7.
4. Facchetti F, Cigognetti M, Fisogni S, et al. Neoplasms derived from plasmacytoid dendritic cells. Mod Pathol 2016;29:98–111.
5. Garnache-Ottou F, Vidal C, Biichle S, et al. How should we diagnose and treat blastic plasmacytoid dendritic cell neoplasm (BPDCN) patients? Blood Adv 2019;3(24):4238–51.
6. Julia F, Dalle S, Duru G, et al. Blastic plasmacytoid dendritic cell neoplasms: clinico-immunohistochemical correlations in a series of 91 patients. Am J Surg Pathol 2014;38:673–80.
7. Leroux D, Mugneret F, Callanan M, et al. CD4(+), CD56(+) DC2 acute leukemia is characterized by recurrent clonal chromosomal changes affecting 6 major targets: a study of 21 cases by the Groupe Français de Cytogénétique Hématologique. Blood 2002;99:4154–9.
8. Pemmaraju N, Lane AA, Sweet KL, et al. Tagraxofusp in blastic plasmacytoid dendritic-cell neoplasm. N Engl J Med 2019;380:1628–37.
9. Reimer P, Rüdiger T, Kraemer D, et al. What is CD4+CD56+ malignancy and how should it be treated? Bone Marrow Transplant 2003;32:637–46.
10. Sapienza MR, Pileri A, Derenzini E, et al. Blastic plasmacytoid dendritic cell neoplasm: state of the art and prospects. Cancers 2019;11 [pii:E595].
11. Taylor J, Haddadin M, Upadhyay VA, et al. Multicenter analysis of outcomes in blastic plasmacytoid dendritic cell neoplasm offers a pre-targeted therapy benchmark. Blood 2019;134(8):678–87.
12. Guru Murthy GS, Pemmaraju N, Atallah E. Epidemiology and survival of blastic plasmacytoid dendritic cell neoplasm. Leuk Res 2018;73:21–3.
13. Kharfan-Dabaja MA, Lazarus HM, Nishihori T, et al. Diagnostic and therapeutic advances in blastic plasmacytoid dendritic cell neoplasm: a focus on hematopoietic cell transplantation. Biol Blood Marrow Transplant 2013;19:1006–12.
14. Laribi K, Denizon N, Besançon A, et al. Blastic plasmacytoid dendritic cell neoplasm: from origin of the cell to targeted therapies. Biol Blood Marrow Transplant 2016;22:1357–67.

15. Pileri SA, Ascani S, Cox MC, et al. Myeloid sarcoma: clinico-pathologic, phenotypic and cytogenetic analysis of 92 adult patients. Leukemia 2007;21:340–50.
16. Tsagarakis NJ, Kentrou NA, Papadimitriou KA, et al. Acute lymphoplasmacytoid dendritic cell (DC2) leukemia: results from the Hellenic Dendritic Cell Leukemia Study Group. Leuk Res 2010;34:438–46.
17. Tzankov A, Hebeda K, Kremer M, et al. Plasmacytoid dendritic cell proliferations and neoplasms involving the bone marrow: summary of the workshop cases submitted to the 18th Meeting of the European Association for Haematopathology (EAHP) organized by the European Bone Marrow Working Group, Basel 2016. Ann Hematol 2017;96:765–77.
18. Venugopal S, Zhou S, El Jamal SM, et al. Blastic plasmacytoid dendritic cell neoplasm-current insights. Clin Lymphoma Myeloma Leuk 2019;19(9):545–54.
19. Jegalian AG, Buxbaum NP, Facchetti F, et al. Blastic plasmacytoid dendritic cell neoplasm in children: diagnostic features and clinical implications. Haematologica 2010;95:1873–9.
20. Amitay-Laish I, Sundram U, Hoppe RT, et al. Localized skin-limited blastic plasmacytoid dendritic cell neoplasm: A subset with possible durable remission without transplantation. JAAD Case Rep 2017;3:310–5.
21. Assaf C, Gellrich S, Steinhoff M, et al. Cutaneous lymphomas in Germany: an analysis of the Central Cutaneous Lymphoma Registry of the German Society of Dermatology (DDG). J Dtsch Dermatol Ges 2007;5:662–8.
22. Bénet C, Gomez A, Aguilar C, et al. Histologic and immunohistologic characterization of skin localization of myeloid disorders: a study of 173 cases. Am J Clin Pathol 2011;135:278–90.
23. Martín-Martín L, López A, Vidriales B, et al. Classification and clinical behavior of blastic plasmacytoid dendritic cell neoplasms according to their maturation-associated immunophenotypic profile. Oncotarget 2015;6:19204–16.
24. Petrella T, Dalac S, Maynadié M, et al. CD4+ CD56+ cutaneous neoplasms: a distinct hematological entity? Groupe Français d'Etude des Lymphomes Cutanés (GFELC). Am J Surg Pathol 1999;23:137–46.
25. Petrella T, Bagot M, Willemze R, et al. Blastic NK-cell lymphomas (agranular CD4+CD56+ hematodermic neoplasms): a review. Am J Clin Pathol 2005;123:662–75.
26. Pileri A, Delfino C, Grandi V, et al. Blastic plasmacytoid dendritic cell neoplasm (BPDCN): the cutaneous sanctuary. G Ital Dermatol Venereol 2012;147:603–8.
27. Barros Romão CMDS, Santos Júnior CJD, Leite LAC, et al. Blastic plasmacytoid dendritic cell neoplasm with pulmonary involvement and atypical skin lesion. Am J Case Rep 2017;18:692–5.
28. Murphy N, Owens D, Hinds E, et al. Blastic plasmacytoid dendritic cell neoplasm (BPDCN) in leukaemic phase without skin lesions: a diagnostic and management challenge. Pathology 2019;51:439–41.
29. Silveira SO, Fernandes CMA, Pinto ÉB, et al. Blastic plasmacytoid dendritic cell neoplasm: an early presentation. Dermatol Online J 2019;25 [pii: 13030/qt9xd132gs].
30. Scarisbrick JJ, Morris S. How big is your hand and should you use it to score skin in cutaneous T-cell lymphoma? Br J Dermatol 2013;169:260–5.
31. Stevens SR, Ke MS, Parry EJ, et al. Quantifying skin disease burden in mycosis fungoides-type cutaneous T-cell lymphomas: the severity-weighted assessment tool (SWAT). Arch Dermatol 2002;138:42–8.
32. Julia F, Petrella T, Beylot-Barry M, et al. Blastic plasmacytoid dendritic cell neoplasm: clinical features in 90 patients. Br J Dermatol 2013;169:579–86.

33. Lee SE, Park HY, Kwon D, et al. Blastic plasmacytoid dendritic cell neoplasm with unusual extracutaneous manifestation: two case reports and literature review. Medicine (Baltimore) 2019;98:e14344.

34. Yu F, Sun K, Wang Z. Atypical presentation of blastic plasmacytoid dendritic cell neoplasm: a potential diagnostic pitfall in nasal cavity. Oral Surg Oral Med Oral Pathol Oral Radiol 2018;126:e212–4.

35. Dornbos D, Elder JB, Otero JJ, et al. Spinal cord toxicity from intrathecal chemotherapy: a case with clinicopathologic correlation. World Neurosurg 2019;128: 381–4.

36. Zheng G, Schmieg J, Guan H, et al. Blastic plasmacytoid dendritic cell neoplasm: cytopathologic findings. Acta Cytol 2012;56:204–8.

37. Fu Y, Fesler M, Mahmud G, et al. Narrowing down the common deleted region of 5q to 6.0 Mb in blastic plasmacytoid dendritic cell neoplasms. Cancer Genet 2013;206:293–8.

38. Kodaira H, Kobayashi S, Shimura H. t(6;8)(p21;q24)in blastic plasmacytoid dendritic cell neoplasma (Sapporo). Presented at the 75th Annual meeting of the Japanese Society of Hematology, 2013.

39. Kubota S, Tokunaga K, Umezu T, et al. Lineage-specific RUNX2 super-enhancer activates MYC and promotes the development of blastic plasmacytoid dendritic cell neoplasm. Nat Commun 2019;10:1653.

40. Momoi A, Toba K, Kawai K, et al. Cutaneous lymphoblastic lymphoma of putative plasmacytoid dendritic cell-precursor origin: two cases. Leuk Res 2002;26: 693–8.

41. Nakamura Y, Kayano H, Kakegawa E, et al. Identification of SUPT3H as a novel 8q24/MYC partner in blastic plasmacytoid dendritic cell neoplasm with t(6;8)(p21;q24) translocation. Blood Cancer J 2015;5:e301.

42. Sakamoto K, Katayama R, Asaka R, et al. Recurrent 8q24 rearrangement in blastic plasmacytoid dendritic cell neoplasm: association with immunoblastoid cytomorphology, MYC expression, and drug response. Leukemia 2018;32:2590–603.

43. Takiuchi Y, Maruoka H, Aoki K, et al. Leukemic manifestation of blastic plasmacytoid dendritic cell neoplasm lacking skin lesion: a borderline case between acute monocytic leukemia. J Clin Exp Hematop 2012;52:107–11.

44. Boddu PC, Wang SA, Pemmaraju N, et al. 8q24/MYC rearrangement is a recurrent cytogenetic abnormality in blastic plasmacytoid dendritic cell neoplasms. Leuk Res 2018;66:73–8.

45. Harley S, Kampagianni O, Lee A, et al. A rare case of blastic plasmacytoid dendritic cell neoplasm with aberrant immunophenotypic profile and unusual cytogenetics. Am J Clin Pathol 2016;146:163.

46. Kurt H, Khoury JD, Medeiros LJ, et al. Blastic plasmacytoid dendritic cell neoplasm with unusual morphology, MYC rearrangement and TET2 and DNMT3A mutations. Br J Haematol 2018;181:305.

47. Sumarriva Lezama L, Chisholm KM, Carneal E, et al. An analysis of blastic plasmacytoid dendritic cell neoplasm with translocations involving the MYC locus identifies t(6;8)(p21;q24) as a recurrent cytogenetic abnormality. Histopathology 2018;73:767–76.

48. Deotare U, Yee KWL, Le LW, et al. Blastic plasmacytoid dendritic cell neoplasm with leukemic presentation: 10-color flow cytometry diagnosis and HyperCVAD therapy. Am J Hematol 2016;91:283–6.

49. Loghavi S, Khoury JD. Disseminated blastic plasmacytoid dendritic cell neoplasm. Blood 2015;126:558.

50. Chamoun K, Loghavi S, Pemmaraju N, et al. Early detection of transformation to BPDCN in a patient with MDS. Exp Hematol Oncol 2018;7:26.
51. Feuillard J, Jacob M-C, Valensi F, et al. Clinical and biologic features of CD4(+) CD56(+) malignancies. Blood 2002;99:1556–63.
52. Alayed K, Patel KP, Konoplev S, et al. TET2 mutations, myelodysplastic features, and a distinct immunoprofile characterize blastic plasmacytoid dendritic cell neoplasm in the bone marrow. Am J Hematol 2013;88:1055–61.
53. Sukswai N, Aung PP, Yin CC, et al. Dual expression of TCF4 and CD123 is highly sensitive and specific for blastic plasmacytoid dendritic cell neoplasm. Am J Surg Pathol 2019;43(10):1429–37.
54. Martín-Martín L, Almeida J, Pomares H, et al. Blastic plasmacytoid dendritic cell neoplasm frequently shows occult central nervous system involvement at diagnosis and benefits from intrathecal therapy. Oncotarget 2016;7:10174–81.
55. Angelot-Delettre F, Biichle S, Ferrand C, et al. Intracytoplasmic detection of TCL1–but not ILT7-by flow cytometry is useful for blastic plasmacytoid dendritic cell leukemia diagnosis. Cytometry A 2012;81:718–24.
56. Boiocchi L, Lonardi S, Vermi W, et al. BDCA-2 (CD303): a highly specific marker for normal and neoplastic plasmacytoid dendritic cells. Blood 2013;122:296–7.
57. Petrella T, Meijer CJLM, Dalac S, et al. TCL1 and CLA expression in agranular CD4/CD56 hematodermic neoplasms (blastic NK-cell lymphomas) and leukemia cutis. Am J Clin Pathol 2004;122:307–13.
58. Djokic M, Björklund E, Blennow E, et al. Overexpression of CD123 correlates with the hyperdiploid genotype in acute lymphoblastic leukemia. Haematologica 2009;94:1016–9.
59. Jordan CT, Upchurch D, Szilvassy SJ, et al. The interleukin-3 receptor alpha chain is a unique marker for human acute myelogenous leukemia stem cells. Leukemia 2000;14:1777–84.
60. Lhermitte L, de Labarthe A, Dupret C, et al. Most immature T-ALLs express Ra-IL3 (CD123): possible target for DT-IL3 therapy. Leukemia 2006;20:1908–10.
61. Garnache-Ottou F, Feuillard J, Ferrand C, et al. Extended diagnostic criteria for plasmacytoid dendritic cell leukaemia. Br J Haematol 2009;145:624–36.
62. Solly F, Angelot F, Garand R, et al. CD304 is preferentially expressed on a subset of B-lineage acute lymphoblastic leukemia and represents a novel marker for minimal residual disease detection by flow cytometry. Cytometry A 2012;81: 17–24.
63. Narducci MG, Pescarmona E, Lazzeri C, et al. Regulation of TCL1 expression in B- and T-cell lymphomas and reactive lymphoid tissues. Cancer Res 2000;60: 2095–100.
64. Cota C, Vale E, Viana I, et al. Cutaneous manifestations of blastic plasmacytoid dendritic cell neoplasm-morphologic and phenotypic variability in a series of 33 patients. Am J Surg Pathol 2010;34:75–87.
65. Garnache-Ottou F, Chaperot L, Biichle S, et al. Expression of the myeloid-associated marker CD33 is not an exclusive factor for leukemic plasmacytoid dendritic cells. Blood 2005;105:1256–64.
66. Kawai K. CD56-negative blastic natural killer-cell lymphoma (agranular CD4(+)/ CD56(+) haematodermic neoplasm)? Br J Dermatol 2005;152:369–70.
67. Lamar E, Roggy A, Le Calvez G, et al. Blastic plasmacytoid dendritic cell neoplasm: report of a case with atypical cytology and immunophenotype. J Blood Disord 2015;2:1033.
68. Montes-Moreno S, Ramos-Medina R, Martínez-López A, et al. SPIB, a novel immunohistochemical marker for human blastic plasmacytoid dendritic cell

neoplasms: characterization of its expression in major hematolymphoid neoplasms. Blood 2013;121:643–7.

69. Khoury JD, Medeiros LJ, Manning JT, et al. CD56(+) TdT(+) blastic natural killer cell tumor of the skin: a primitive systemic malignancy related to myelomonocytic leukemia. Cancer 2002;94:2401–8.

70. Vermi W, Facchetti F, Rosati S, et al. Nodal and extranodal tumor-forming accumulation of plasmacytoid monocytes/interferon-producing cells associated with myeloid disorders. Am J Surg Pathol 2004;28:585–95.

71. Vitte F, Fabiani B, Bénet C, et al. Specific skin lesions in chronic myelomonocytic leukemia: a spectrum of myelomonocytic and dendritic cell proliferations: a study of 42 cases. Am J Surg Pathol 2012;36:1302–16.

72. Swerdlow SH, Campo E, Harris NL, et al. WHO classification of tumours of haematopoietic and lymphoid tissues. Lyon (France): International Agency for Research on Cancer; 2017.

73. Lucas N, Duchmann M, Rameau P, et al. Biology and prognostic impact of clonal plasmacytoid dendritic cells in chronic myelomonocytic leukemia. Leukemia 2019;33(10):2466–80.

74. Hamadeh F, Awadallah A, Meyerson HJ, et al. Flow cytometry identifies a spectrum of maturation in myeloid neoplasms having plasmacytoid dendritic cell differentiation. Cytometry B Clin Cytom 2020;98(1):43–51.

Blastic Plasmacytoid Dendritic Cell Neoplasm

The Dermatologist's Perspective

Jesse P. Hirner, MD, John T. O'Malley, MD, PhD,
Nicole R. LeBoeuf, MD, MPH*

KEYWORDS

- Blastic plasmacytoid dendritic cell neoplasm • BPDCN
- CD4$^+$CD56$^+$ hematodermic neoplasm • Blastic natural-killer cell lymphoma

KEY POINTS

- Blastic plasmacytoid dendritic cell neoplasm (BPDCN) commonly involves the skin, and cutaneous involvement is often the presenting sign.
- BPDCN may present as deep purple or brown patches, plaques, or nodules in a localized or disseminated pattern and may involve mucous membranes.
- Skin biopsy is often the key to diagnosis. When possible, the clinician should alert the pathologist to the clinical possibility of BPDCN, because specialized immunohistochemical stains are used to make the definitive diagnosis.

INTRODUCTION

Blastic plasmacytoid dendritic cell neoplasm (BPDCN) is a rare, aggressive malignancy of plasmacytoid dendritic cells (pDCs).[1] pDCs are a bone marrow–derived cell line found primarily in the lymphoid tissue and circulation.[2] In normal, healthy skin, pDCs are rare or absent.[2] In select skin diseases, such as psoriasis, contact dermatitis, and lupus erythematosus, they are recruited to the skin, where they produce type I interferons (IFNs), IFN-α and IFN-β, and help regulate the immune response.[2–5] In addition to inflammatory skin conditions, they play an important role in early antiviral immune responses and wound healing[2–5]; pDCs recognize microbial nucleic acids via intracellular Toll-like receptor 7 (TLR7) and TLR8, which trigger expression of IFNs.

BPDCN has previously been termed CD4$^+$CD56$^+$ hematodermic neoplasm and blastic natural-killer cell lymphoma.[1] In the 2008 World Health Organization (WHO) classification of myeloid neoplasms and leukemia, BPDCN was classified

Department of Dermatology, The Center For Cutaneous Oncology, Dana-Farber Cancer Institute, Brigham and Women's Hospital, Harvard Medical School, 375 Longwood Avenue, Boston, MA 02115, USA
* Corresponding author.
E-mail address: Nleboeuf@bwh.harvard.edu

Hematol Oncol Clin N Am 34 (2020) 501–509
https://doi.org/10.1016/j.hoc.2020.01.001
0889-8588/20/© 2020 Elsevier Inc. All rights reserved.

under acute myeloid leukemia and related neoplasms. In the 2016 WHO categorization, BPDCN is classified into its own category among myeloproliferative neoplasms. The incidence of BPDCN is approximately 0.4 cases per 100,000 individuals.[6] BPDCN has a male predominance with reported male:female ratios ranging from (1.9:1–4:1).[6–10] Most patients are white, and it primarily affects older adults with a mean age of 58 to 71.[6–11] The skin is the most common non–bone marrow organ involved and often precedes bone marrow involvement.[7,8,11] Thus, skin involvement is commonly the initial presenting sign of the disease, and skin biopsy is often the key in making the diagnosis.[7,11] Diagnosis of BPDCN is often delayed because of diagnostic pitfalls; it may be misdiagnosed as acute myelogenous leukemia cutis, or if there are one or a few lesions, it may initially be mistaken for traumatic purpura. Mortality is high; survival is short, and early recognition of this disease is increasingly important given the availability of effective targeted treatment of the interleukin-3 (IL-3)/IL-3R pathway, important in the pathogenesis of BPDCN.[6,12] It is important for dermatologists and oncologists to be familiar with the cutaneous manifestations of BPDCN to help facilitate early diagnosis, systemic workup, and treatment of these patients.

CUTANEOUS MANIFESTATIONS OF BLASTIC PLASMACYTOID DENDRITIC CELL NEOPLASM

BPDCN presents as deep purple or brown patches, plaques, or tumors on the skin.[7,11] In the largest study on the clinical presentation of BPDCN, which retrospectively reviewed 90 patients, 73% presented with 1 or a few nodules, 14% with disseminated plaques, and 12% with bruiselike patches.[7] In a retrospective analysis of 33 patients, disseminated plaques or nodules were most frequently represented.[11] As such, BPDCN may be limited to a single location, or widely disseminated (**Figs. 1–4**). Localized disease may occur on the trunk, head and neck, or extremities, and it is not clear that 1 location is more commonly affected than others; the authors' institutional experience and review of cases in the literature suggest the head, upper trunk, and upper extremities are more commonly involved than the lower trunk and extremities. Disseminated disease commonly affects all 3 sites, but the lesions are typically most dense on the upper trunk. Patients with disseminated skin involvement at diagnosis are more likely to have detectable systemic disease than patients with more limited skin disease, but the extent of skin disease does not appear to correlate with survival.[7] In most cases, BPDCN appears first in the skin and may be the only organ involved initially. Eventually, rapid leukemic spread and multiorgan involvement occur, including the bone marrow (34%–87% of cases) and lymph nodes (41%–52% of cases).[6,7,9,10,13] In approximately 10% of the cases, leukemic involvement may occur in the absence of skin disease.[14–23]

Skin tropism of the neoplastic cells of BPDCN is thought to be secondary to the surface expression of skin-migration molecules, such as cutaneous lymphocyte-associated antigen, one of the E-selectin ligands, which binds to E-selectin on high-endothelial venules.[2] In addition, the local cutaneous microenvironment of chemokines binding CXCR3, CXCR4, CCR6, or CCR7 expressed by the neoplastic cells likely contributes to skin-homing.[2,15] However, the exact mechanisms underlying the cutaneous tropism have not been fully elucidated.

Mucosal lesions reportedly occur in a minority of patients, but may be underreported.[2] Mucosal disease typically appears similar to cutaneous disease with deep purple macules, papules, or nodules (**Fig. 5**).[7]

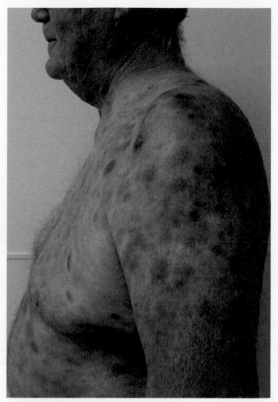

Fig. 1. Violaceous, round, confluent plaques of BPDCN on the trunk, arms, and face. BPDCN may be disseminated, as in this case, or localized.

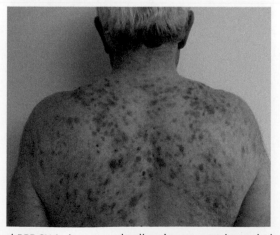

Fig. 2. Disseminated BPDCN in brown and yellow-brown papules and plaques.

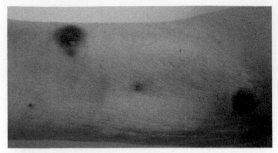

Fig. 3. Deep purple localized BPDCN on the arm.

DIFFERENTIAL DIAGNOSIS

The initial clinical differential diagnosis for BPDCN depends on the clinical presentation, extent, and thickness of lesions and includes common traumatic ecchymoses, purpuric disorders, angiosarcoma, Kaposi sarcoma, neuroblastoma, vascular metastases, extramedullary hematopoiesis, and skin involvement by hematologic neoplasms other than BPDCN.

BIOPSY APPROACH AND HISTOPATHOLOGIC FEATURES

Skin biopsies are the key to making the diagnosis and should include deep dermis and, ideally, some subcutaneous fat. For punch, incisional, or small macules or

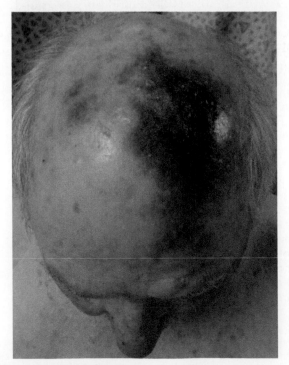

Fig. 4. A focal plaque of BPDCN infiltration on the scalp.

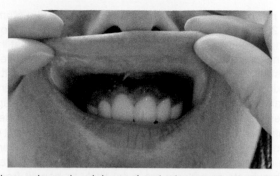

Fig. 5. Deep purple papules and nodules on the gingiva representing BPDCN of the mucosa.

papules, excisional biopsy should be performed. Shave biopsy should be avoided. Dermatologists should alert the pathologist that BPDCN is in the clinical differential diagnosis when possible, because uncommonly used immunohistochemical (IHC) stains are needed to make the diagnosis, and it may be histologically mistaken for acute myelogenous leukemia cutis. BPDCN is characterized by a dense dermal monomorphous infiltrate of medium-sized blastoid cells with small or absent nucleoli.[11,24] BPDCN's IHC phenotype is typified by expression of CD4, CD56, CD123, CD303 (BDCA2), TCL-1, and BCL-2.[7,24,25] The first five, which are perhaps the most specific markers, are all simultaneously expressed in only 46% of patients.[25] Positivity for four of the five may be used to make the diagnosis.[11] CD303 expression and high Ki-67 expression have been associated with improved survival.[25] Some studies have found terminal deoxynucleotidyltransferase negativity in BPDCN cells begets worse outcomes, but study data on this are conflicting.[6,8,25]

EVALUATION AND PROGNOSIS OF THE BLASTIC PLASMACYTOID DENDRITIC CELL NEOPLASM PATIENT

Initial staging evaluation includes hematologic evaluation, bone marrow biopsy, and imaging to assess for leukemic, nodal, and visceral involvement. The lymph nodes, bone marrow, and blood appear to be the most commonly involved extracutaneous sites.[6,8,11,25] At the time of initial presentation, 27% to 87% of patients will have detectable bone marrow involvement; 22% to 28% will have detectable blood involvement, and 6% to 41% will have lymph node involvement.[6–9,11,13] Associated myeloid disorders, including chronic myelogenous leukemia and myelodysplastic syndrome, have been reported.[7] Pediatric patients have a greater 5-year overall survival (OS) than older patients, and OS worsens with increasing age.[6,8,26] Extent of skin involvement and presence of systemic involvement at presentation do not seem to be strong predictors of survival. Julia and colleagues,[7] in a retrospective analysis of 90 patients, found that type of skin disease did not predict survival. Specifically, presence of nodular lesions or disseminated skin involvement was not adverse prognostic factors compared with macular lesions limited to "1 or 2 body areas."[7] Suzuki and colleagues,[24] in a retrospective analysis including 35 BPDCN patients, found a trend toward decreased survival in patients with disseminated disease compared with patients with nodular disease, but it did not reach statistical significance. Two studies, totaling 149 patients, reported that results of initial staging evaluation did not correlate with survival, and presence of systemic involvement did not predict decreased survival.[7,8] Aoki and colleagues[9] found that the presence of marrow involvement at presentation did not predict survival in patients who received a stem cell transplant (SCT). Eleven of 25 patients in this study were treated with autologous SCT, and 14 were treated with allogeneic SCT. Cota and colleagues[11] report that in a retrospective study of 33 patients, skin-limited disease had a trend toward improved survival, but it did not reach statistical significance. Cumulatively, these results suggest that morphology of skin lesion, extent of skin involvement, and initial staging were not useful prognostic markers, and to date, the disease remains uniformly aggressive. However, these studies were published before the advent of newer targeted therapies; the number of patients was limited, and all 4 studies were retrospective. It is important that future studies continue to address whether early treatment with the targeted therapies impacts disease course, which approaches best deplete disease across compartments and which subsets of patients are most likely to benefit from early targeted or combination therapy.

BLASTIC PLASMACYTOID DENDRITIC CELL NEOPLASM TREATMENT

Increased understanding of the oncogenomic landscape and pathogenesis of BPDCN has resulted in development of targeted therapies that have shown efficacy above standard chemotherapy regimens. The interleukin-3 receptor alpha subunit, also known as CD123, is overexpressed in BPDCN. Tagraxofusp, an interleukin-3–truncated diphtheria toxin conjugate, is approved by the Food and Drug Administration and, in the authors' experience, results in rapid clearance of skin nodules, often leaving postinflammatory hyperpigmentation (**Fig. 6**).[12] Biopsy may be required to determine if there is residual BPDCN that has regressed but not resolved, or only pigmentary alteration. Azacytidine, a DNA methyltransferase inhibitor, may be used to overcome tagraxofusp resistance by restoring lost activity in the diphthamide synthesis pathway.[27] BPDCN is BCL-2 dependent, and venetoclax has been used with rapid clearance of skin lesions in a subset of patients.[28] Although traditional cytotoxic chemotherapy can also be used, allogeneic SCT during first complete remission can provide long-term remission for some patients.[9,10,29,30] There does not appear to be a survival difference between SCT recipients who received reduced intensity or non-myeloablative conditioning regimens and those who received myeloablative conditioning.[9,10,30] Based on the authors' dermatologic oncology experience with

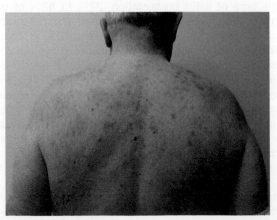

Fig. 6. Brown macules and patches at the site of prior BPDCN skin lesions in a patient treated with tagraxofusp with response and residual hyperpigmentation.

allogeneic SCT in cutaneous lymphoma, total skin electron beam has been used at the authors' institution as part of transplant conditioning for BPDCN, with the goal of eliminating additional subclinical disease burden at the time of SCT.[31–33] Determination of outcomes from this approach is pending long-term follow-up. In summary, the goal of care for BPDCN patients is allogeneic SCT after induction of the first complete remission, ideally confirmed with skin biopsy to confirm complete response in all compartments; the optimal combination of the aforementioned therapies continues to be explored to maximize the chances of long-term remission from this aggressive malignancy.

SUMMARY

BPDCN is a rare, aggressive malignancy that commonly presents on the skin. It most commonly presents as deep purple or brown patches, plaques, or nodules and may present in a disseminated or localized distribution. Skin biopsy is often the key to diagnosis. Although lack of systemic involvement at presentation may seem reassuring, the disease presents without extracutaneous sites 31% to 61% of the time, and survival is poor regardless of presentation.[7,11] Delays in diagnosis, referral, treatment, and transplant should all be avoided. In addition to oncologists, dermatologists have an important role in assuring accurate and timely diagnosis of this aggressive disease, and familiarity with its presentation will aid in appropriate and expedited treatment.

REFERENCES

1. Petrella T, Comeau MR, Maynadie M, et al. Agranular CD4+ CD56+ hematodermic neoplasm (blastic NK-cell lymphoma) originates from a population of CD56+ precursor cells related to plasmacytoid monocytes. Am J Surg Pathol 2002;26(7): 852–62.

2. Sozzani S, Vermi W, Del Prete A, et al. Trafficking properties of plasmacytoid dendritic cells in health and disease. Trends Immunol 2010;31(7):270–7.

3. Wollenberg A, Wagner M, Gunther S, et al. Plasmacytoid dendritic cells: a new cutaneous dendritic cell subset with distinct role in inflammatory skin diseases. J Invest Dermatol 2002;119(5):1096–102.

4. Guiducii C, Tripodo C, Gong M, et al. Autoimmune skin inflammation is dependent on plasmacytoid dendritic cell activation by nucleic acids via TLR7 and TLR9. J Exp Med 2010;207(13):2931–42.

5. Gregorio J, Meller S, Conrad C, et al. Plasmacytoid dendritic cells sense skin injury and promote wound healing through type I interferons. J Exp Med 2010; 2017(13):2921–30.

6. Guru Murthy GS, Pemmaraju N, Attallah E. Epidemiology and survival of blastic plasmacytoid dendritic cell neoplasm. Leuk Res 2018;73:21–3.

7. Julia F, Petrella T, Beylot-Barry M, et al. Blastic plasmacytoid dendritic cell neoplasm: clinical features in 90 patients. Br J Dermatol 2012;169(3):579–86.

8. Taylor J, Haddadin M, Updadhyay VA, et al. Multicenter analysis of outcomes in blastic plasmacytoid dendritic cell neoplasm offers a pretargeted therapy benchmark. Blood 2019;134(8):678–87.

9. Aoki T, Suzuki R, Kuwatsuka Y, et al. Long-term survival following autologous and allogeneic stem cell transplantation for blastic plasmacytoid dendritic cell neoplasm. Blood 2015;125(23):3559–62.

10. Kharfan-Dabaja MA, Al Malki MM, Deotare U, et al. Haematopoietic cell transplantation for blastic plasmacytoid dendritic cell neoplasm: a North American multicentre collaborative study. Br J Haematol 2017;179(5):781–9.

11. Cota C, Vale E, Viana I, et al. Cutaneous manifestations of blastic plasmacytoid dendritic cell neoplasm–morphologic and phenotypic variability in a series of 33 patients. Am J Surg Pathol 2010;34(1):75–87.

12. Pemmeraju N, Lane AA, Sweet KL, et al. Tagraxofusp in blastic plasmacytoid dendritic-cell neoplasm. N Engl J Med 2019;380(17):1628–37.

13. Feuillard J, Jacob M, Valensi F, et al. Clinical and biological features of $CD4^+CD56^+$ malignancies. Blood 2002;99(5):1556–63.

14. Murphy N, Owens D, Hinds E, et al. Blastic plasmacytoid dendritic cell neoplasm (BPDCN) in leukaemic phase without skin lesions: a diagnostic and management challenge. Pathology 2019;51(4):439–41.

15. Sapienza MR, Pileri A, Derenzini E, et al. Blastic plasmacytoid dendritic cell neoplasm: state of the art and prospects. Cancer 2019;11(5):E595.

16. Endo K, Mihara K, Oiwa H, et al. Lung involvement at the initial presentation in blastic plasmacytoid dendritic cell neoplasm lacking cutaneous lesion. Ann Hematol 2013;92(2):269–70.

17. Pagano L, Valentini CG, Pulsoni A, et al. Blastic plasmacytoid dendritic cell neoplasm with leukemic presentation: an Italian multicenter study. Haematologica 2013;98(2):239–46.

18. Paluri R, Nabell L, Borak S, et al. Unique presentation of blastic plasmacytoid dendritic cell neoplasm: a single-center experience and literature review. Hematol Oncol 2015;33(4):206–11.

19. Rauh MJ, Rahman F, Good D, et al. Blastic plasmacytoid dendritic cell neoplasm with leukemic presentation, lacking cutaneous involvement: case series and literature review. Leuk Res 2012;36(1):82–6.

20. Wang H, Cao J, Hong X. Blastic plasmacytoid dendritic cell neoplasm without cutaneous lesion at presentation: case report and literature review. Acta Hematol 2012;127(2):124–7.

21. Facchetti F, Cigognetti M, Fisogni S, et al. Neoplasms derived from plasmacytoid dendritic cells. Mod Pathol 2016;29(2):98–111.

22. Bendriss-Vermare N, Chaperot L, Peoc'h M, et al. In situ leukemic plasmacytoid dendritic cell pattern of chemokine receptors expression and in vitro migratory response. Leukemia 2004;18(9):1491–8.

23. Patrella T, Comeau MR, Maynadie M, et al. Agranular CD4+CD56+ hematodermic neoplasms (blastic NK-cell lymphoma) originates from a population of CD56+ precursor cells related to plasmacytoid monocytes. Am J Surg Pathol 2002;26(7):852–62.

24. Suzuki Y, Kato S, Kohno K, et al. Clinicopathological analysis of 46 cases of CD4+ and/or CD56+ immature haematolymphoid malignancy: reappraisal of blastic plasmacytoid dendritic cell and related neoplasms. Histopathology 2017;71(6):972–84.

25. Julia F, Dalle S, Duru G, et al. Blastic plasmacytoid dendritic cell neoplasms: clinico-immunohistochemical correlations in a series of 91 patients. Am J Surg Pathol 2014;38(5):673–80.

26. Kim MJ, Nasr H, Kabir B, et al. Pediatric blastic plasmacytoid dendritic cell neoplasm: a systematic literature review. J Pediatr Hematol Oncol 2017;39(7): 528–37.

27. Togami K, Pastika T, Stephansky J, et al. DNA methyltransferase inhibition overcomes diphthamide pathway deficiencies underlying CD123-targeted treatment resistance. J Clin Invest 2019;129(11):5005–19.
28. Montero J, Stephansky J, Cai T, et al. Blastic plasmacytoid dendritic cell neoplasm is dependent on BCL2 and sensitive to venetoclax. Cancer Discov 2017;7(2):156–64.
29. Heinicke T, Hutten H, Kalinski T, et al. Sustained remission of blastic plasmacytoid dendritic cell neoplasm after unrelated allogeneic stem cell transplantation–a single center experience. Ann Hematol 2015;94(2):283–7.
30. Leclerc M, Peffault R, Michallet M, et al. Can a reduced-intensity conditioning regimen cure blastic plasmacytoid dendritic cell neoplasm. Blood 2017;129(9): 1227–30.
31. Duvic M, Donato M, Dabaja B, et al. Total skin electron beam and non-myeloablative allogeneic hematopoietic stem cell transplantation in advanced mycosis fungoides and Sezary syndrome. J Clin Oncol 2010;28(14):2365–72.
32. National Comprehensive Cancer Network. Primary cutaneous lymphomas (version 2.2019). Available at: https://www.nccn.org/professionals/physician_gls/pdf/primary_cutaneous.pdf. Accessed October 24, 2019.
33. Trautinger F, Eder J, Assaf C, et al. European Organization for the Research and Treatment of Cancer consensus recommendations for the treatment of mycosis fungoides/Sezary syndrome–update 2017. Eur J Cancer 2017;77:57–74.

Molecular Features of Blastic Plasmacytoid Dendritic Cell Neoplasm
DNA Mutations and Epigenetics

Maria Rosaria Sapienza, MS, PhD*, Stefano Pileri, MD, PhD

KEYWORDS

- Blastic plasmacytoid dendritic cell neoplasm (BPDCN) • Epigenetics • Methylation
- BRD4 • Azacitidine • NGS

KEY POINTS

- Blastic plasmacytoid dendritic cell neoplasm (BPDCN) displays a DNA mutational spectrum typically myeloid, with recurrent mutations of epigenetic modifiers, transcriptional regulators, and splicing factors.
- The epigenetic modifier gene mutations are the most frequent gene mutations and induce profound alterations of the epigenetic program.
- BPDCN epigenetic vulnerability is a promising target for epigenetic-based therapies.

INTRODUCTION

Blastic plasmacytoid dendritic cell neoplasm (BPDCN) is a rare and aggressive hematologic tumor derived from the malignant transformation of plasmacytoid dendritic cell precursors (pDCs).[1] Its cellular derivation has been controversial and has produced a long history of misdiagnosis and irregular nomenclature, including CD56[+]/TdT[+] blastic NK cell tumor and CD4[+]/CD56[+] hematodermic neoplasm.[2,3] Finally, in 2008, based on the immunophenotypic profile, BPDCN has been classified as a myeloid neoplasm of pDCs derivation.[4,5]

Since then, the number of molecular studies on BPDCN has been growing. The advent of next-generation sequencing (NGS) techniques has rapidly expanded the understanding of BPDCN biology, improved its diagnostic accuracy, and provided novel therapeutic options. More specifically, studies of DNA sequencing have revealed that the BPDCN is a neoplasm recurrently mutated in epigenetic pathway genes, in line with its myeloid derivation.

Division of Diagnostic Haematopathology, European Institute of Oncology, IRCCS, Via Ripamonti 435, Milan 20141, Italy
* Corresponding author.
E-mail addresses: mariarosaria.sapienza@ieo.it; mariarosaria.sapienza@gmail.com

Hematol Oncol Clin N Am 34 (2020) 511–521
https://doi.org/10.1016/j.hoc.2020.01.002
0889-8588/20/© 2020 Elsevier Inc. All rights reserved.

DNA MUTATIONS

The first work on the genetic mutations of BPDCN (**Table 1**) dates back to 2011: the myeloid origin of BPDCN was recently declared and *TET2* mutations were recurrently detected in various myeloid malignancies, including myelodysplastic syndromes (MDS), chronic myelomonocytic leukemia (CMML), or secondary acute myeloid leukemia (AML).[6] Thus, to better confirm at the molecular level the lineage derivation of BPDCN, Jardin and colleagues[7] investigated the mutational status of *TET2* in 13 BPDCNs, by polymerase chain reaction (PCR) assay and direct sequencing. Almost half of the cases (6/13, 54%) presented *TET2* mutations, prevalently frameshift and nonsense, with possible impairment of protein function, as described in other myeloid malignancies. Notably, 4 cases were both *TET2* and *TP53* mutated, suggesting a synergistic effect between the 2 genes.

In keeping with this hypothesis, 1 case carrying *TET2* mutations at diagnosis acquired *TP53* mutations at relapse, further supporting the suspicion of a genetic collaborative interaction. Globally, Jardin and colleagues[7] provided the preliminary evidence of *TET2* involvement in BPDCN pathogenesis.

Next-Generation Sequencing

Advances in NGS have significantly broadened the spectrum and frequency of mutations in BPDCN. Characterization of the BPDCN genomic landscape has led to the

Table 1		
DNA mutational analysis of blastic plasmacytoid dendritic cell neoplasm		
Authors, Reference	**Technique**	**DNA Mutated Genes**
Jardin et al,[7] 2011	aCGH/SNP	*TET2 TP53*
Alayed et al,[8] 2013	PCR assay/TS	*TET2*
Taylor et al,[9] 2013	TS	*TET2, TP53, ASXL1, IDH2, KRAS, ABL1, ARID1A, GNA13, U2AF1, SRSF2, IRF8, ZRSR2*
Menezes et al,[12] 2014	WES/TS	*DNMT3A, IDH1, IDH2, TET1, TE2, ASXL1, ATRX, EZH2, KRAS, NRAS, ETV6, HOXB9, IKZF1, IKZF2, IKZF3, RUNX1, ZEB2, SF3B1, SRSF2, U2AF1, ZRSR2, NPM1, FLT3, FLT3-ID, JAK2, KIT, TP53, CBLB, CBLC, UBE2G2*
Stenzinger et al,[14] 2014	TS	*NRAS, ATM, MET, KRAS, IDH2, KIT, APC, RB1, VHL, BRAF, MLH1, TP53, RET*
Emadali et al,[16] 2016	TS	*ASXL1, EZH2*
Togami et al,[11] 2016	WES/TS	*ZRSR2, SRSF2, SF3B1, U2AF1, SF3A2, SF3B4, TET2, ASXL1, TP53, GNB1, NRAS, IDH2, ETV6, DNMT3A, RUNX1, CRIPAK, NEFH, HNF1A, PAX3, SSC5D*
Sapienza et al,[17] 2019	WES/TS	*ARID1A, CHD8, SMARCA5, SMARCAD1, SMARCD1, TET2, IDH2, ASH1L, ASXL1, ASXL3, MLL2, MLL3, MLL4, SETMAR, SUZ12, KDM4D, PHF2, EP300, EP400, MYST3, MYST4, PHC1, PHC2, EYA2, SRCAP, NRAS, KRAS, BRCA1, ATM, ATR, RAD52, ZRSR2, RET, MAPK1, BRAF, RUNX2, SYK, WNT10, WNT7B, BCL9L, WNT3.*
Ladikou et al,[23] 2018	TS	*TET2, RHOA*
Szczepaniak et al,[24] 2019	TS	*ASXL1, TET2, NF1*

Abbreviation: TS, targeted sequencing.

identification of recurrent mutations in several previously uncharacterized genes. The classes of genes investigated included transcription factors, kinases, cell-cycle regulators, spliceosome genes, and epigenetic regulators, as reported in **Table 1**.

In 2013, Alayed and colleagues[8] sequenced 5 BPDCN cases by a custom-designed panel that was interrogating the entire coding sequences of 28 leukemia-related genes (*ABL1, ASXL1, BRAF, DNMT3A, FGFR, EZH2, FLT3, GATA1, GATA2, HRAS, IDH1, IDH2, IKZF2, JAK2, KIT, KRAS, MDM2, MLL, MPL, MYD88, NOTCH1, NPM1, NRAS, PTPN11, RUNX1, TET2, TP53,* and *WT1*). Apart from *TET2*, none of the remaining 27 genes were mutated. All cases but one presented single or multiple *TET2* mutations, exclusively clustered in exons 3 and 11. In conclusion, Alayed and colleagues[8] confirmed that *TET2* was frequently mutated in BPDCN.

Taylor and colleagues[9] analyzed 7 BPDCN cases by a targeted-sequencing panel of 219 hematologic-related genes and presented the study results in 2013 at the Annual Meeting of the American Society of Hematology. Jardin's molecular findings were restated, with 4/7 and 1/7 patients mutated in *TET2* and *TP53* genes, respectively. The BPDCN cases globally reflected the mutational spectrum of other myeloid neoplasms with mutations of *ASXL1, ARID1A,* and *IDH2* epigenetic modifier genes, *U2AF1* and *SRSF2* splicing factor genes, and with mutations of *ABL1, GNA13,* and *KRAS* genes. Of note, they also found mutated the Interferon regulatory factor gene, *IRF8,* which plays a central role in the differentiation of hematopoietic progenitor cells and, especially, in the proliferation of common dendritic cell precursors.[10] However, the most relevant discovery made by Taylor and colleagues was the recurrence of mutations affecting the *ZRSR2* splicing factor gene in the 4/7 BPDCN cases. Next, the mutational status of the *ZRSR2* gene was extended to a set of additional 32 BPDCN cases and, collectively, as many as 15/39 patients (38.5%) resulted to be *ZRSR2* mutated. All the *ZRSR2* mutations detected were predicted to be highly damaging (frameshift, splice site, or premature stop codon mutations), with probable loss of function of the encoded protein. In BPDCN patients, *ZRSR2* were approximately 10-fold more recurrent than in MDS and AML and correlated to age $\geq$65 ($P = .068$) and male sex ($P = .007$) but not to the clinical outcome. Therefore, *ZRSR2* do not have a prognostic value in BPDCN but, as demonstrated in vivo by Taylor and colleagues, may exert a pathogenic role; mouse models engrafted with BPDCN tumor cells harboring *ZRSR2* with premature stop codon mutation rapidly developed leukemia by retention of the *ZRSR2* mutation. The contribution to BPDCN growth of *ZRSR2* and splicing factors more in general would also be deepened by Togami and colleagues[11] (see later discussion).

Menezes and colleagues[12] performed the first whole-exome sequencing (WES) on a discovery set of 3 BPDCN cases, whose molecular findings were then extensively explored in a validation cohort of 25 cases by a targeted sequencing approach. They used a panel of 38 selected genes, divided into 9 categories: DNA methylation, chromatin remodeling, transcription factors, splicing machinery, protein kinase activity and ubiquitination, 1 nucleophosmin gene, 2 *RAS* family genes, and 1 tumor suppressor gene. Twenty-nine of 38 investigated genes were mutated, and among them, *TET2* was the most frequently mutated gene (36%), followed by *ASXL1* (32%), *NRAS* (20%), *NPM1* (20%), the *IKAROS* family (20%), and *ZEB2* (16%). Only 1 case was *JAK2* or *FLT3-ITD* mutated, at a much lower frequency than AML or myeloproliferative disorders. Overall, almost half of the patients reported mutations of genes involved in either the DNA methylation or chromatin remodeling pathways, and these patients experienced a worse clinical outcome than the unmutated patients. Apart from the epigenetic pathway genes, *IKAROS* family genes were also found recurrently mutated in BPDCN. As is well known, *IKZF1* regulates dendritic cell hematopoiesis, and in the mouse model, its deficiency correlates with reduced production of interferon-α and tumor necrosis factor by plasmacytoid dendritic cells.[13] About 20% of BPDCN cases analyzed carried out mutations of *IKAROS* family genes whose role in BPDCN tumorigenesis remained to be elucidated.

The same year, in 2014, Stenzinger and colleagues[14] investigated 33 BPDCN samples by a targeted sequencing panel of 50 common cancer genes and identified mutations in *NRAS* (27.3% of cases), *ATM* (21.2%), *MET, KRAS, IDH2, KIT* (9.1% each), *APC*, and *RB1* (6.1% each), as well as in *VHL, BRAF, MLH1, TP53*, and *RET* (3% each). Almost all the cases were mutated (29/33) in at least one of the interrogated genes, *NRAS* and *ATM* being the most frequently affected. The only genes belonging to the epigenetic pathway and included in the analysis were *IDH1, IDH2*, and *EZH2*, but only *IDH2* was mutated. *RAS* signaling was the most affected pathway with *NRAS* and *KRAS* showing mutually exclusive mutations. Globally, 35% of BPDCNs were mutated in *RAS* signaling genes, a percentage higher than in other hematologic neoplasms known to harbor *RAS* mutations, such as juvenile myelomonocytic leukemia, CMML, and AML.[15] Thanks to this study, the relevance of *RAS* signaling in BPDCN was underlined.

Emadali and colleagues[16] performed molecular cytogenetic analyses of 46 BPDCN cases and identified recurrent deletions of the *NR3C1* gene (28% of cases). *NR3C1* encodes for a glucocorticoid receptor whose deletion in BPDCN was associated with corticoresistance, dismal prognosis, and a transcriptional signature of *EZH2* loss of function. Subsequently, *NR3C1, ASXL1*, and *EZH2* genes were examined by targeted sequencing to check if their mutational status could be responsible for the *EZH2* dysfunction, but the sequencing results excluded their direct involvement. The role of *N3RC1* glucocorticoid receptor was further explored by connections with transcriptomic and epigenetic information, as detailed in the paragraph "Epigenetics."

Togami and colleagues[11] performed a study on BPDCN based on the WES of 12 cases, targeted sequencing of 24 cases, RNA sequencing of 12 cases and 6 patient-derived xenografts, and single RNA sequencing versus normal plasmacytoid dendritic cells. Genes already described in BPDCN and in other blood cancers, such as *TET2, ASXL1, TP53, GNB1, NRAS, IDH2, ETV6, DNMT3A*, and *RUNX1*, were detected as recurrently mutated, but also novel genes never described before, such as *CRIPAK, NEFH, HNF1A, PAX3*, and *SSC5D*, which may be unique to BPDCN.

Of note, in line with the previous work of Taylor and colleagues,[9] RNA splicing factor genes were very frequently mutated, in as many as 16/24 cases (7 *ZRSR2*, 6 *SRSF2*, 1 each *SF3B1, U2AF1, SF3A2*, and *SF3B4*). The role of *ZRSR2* loss-of-function mutations in the BPDCN pathogenesis was better investigated, and finally, it was demonstrated that the cases *ZRSR2* mutated, compared with the unmutated ones, presented aberrant RNA splicing, with irregular intron retention. In conclusion, Togami and colleagues[11] showed that in BPDCN the frequent mutations of splicing factor genes, and above all *ZRSR2*, may be accountable for the impairment of RNA splicing, defective assembly of gene transcripts, and alteration of pathways central for pDCs maturation and tumor transformation.

Sapienza and colleagues[17] used the WES technique to study 14 BPDCN cases and the CAL1-1 BPDCN cell line. The employment of a sequencing approach, not limiting the investigation to a priori selected genes, allowed the authors to explore the mutational status of the maximum number possible of epigenetic modifier genes and to recognize, as mutated, epigenetic factors never related to BPDCN, like *PHF2* histone demethylase, an enhancer of the TP53-tumor suppressor activity,[18] and Chromodomain helicase DNA-binding protein-8, *CHD8* gene, a positive regulator of the *E2F*-dependent transcription and cell-cycle progression.[19]

Globally, 25 epigenetic pathway genes controlling either chromatin accessibility, DNA methylation, or histone posttranscriptional modifications (methylation, demethylation, acetylation, ubiquitination, dephosphorylation, and exchange) have been found mutated. Most of the mutations clustered in the histone methylation pathway, specifically in genes belonging to the Polycomb repressive complex 2 (PRC2) (*ASXL1, ASXL3, SUZ12*) and in histone methyltransferases (*ASHL1, SETMAR, MLL*), possibly compromise the integrity of the methylation program at both DNA and histone levels. Of note, 12/14 BPDCN cases (86%) harbored at least 1 of the 25 mutated epigenetic pathway genes, and more than half of cases (57.14%) reported a potentially deleterious mutation. Besides the epigenetic pathway, mutations affecting programs common to other myeloid malignancies, such as the DNA repair process,[20] Wnt/β-catenin signaling,[21] and the differentiation pathway, were also identified.[22] However, the epigenetic biological process resulted to be the most critically compromised by recurrent and damaging mutations.

Of interest, the exome mutational findings, integrated with RNA and chromatin immunoprecipitation (ChIP)-sequencing data, helped to discover new epigenetic traits of BPDCN, discussed later, in the paragraph entitled "Epigenetics"

Ladikou and colleagues[23] carried out the targeted sequencing of hot-spot mutations on 12 genes, from the circulating free DNA of 1 BPDCN patient. At diagnosis, they detected a single frameshift mutation of *TET2* and a missense mutation of *RHOA* gene. DNA targeted sequencing at the second time point, after the development of acute leukemic disease, demonstrated changes to the mutational frequency; although the *RHOA* mutation was undetectable, the *TET2* mutation was notably increased. This finding suggested that the acute leukemic phase could be associated with either (i) a single clone, both *TET2* and *RHOA* mutated, that loses the *RHOA* mutation during the tumor evolution; or (ii) 2 clones, 1 *TET2* and the other *RHOA* mutated. In the latter hypothesis, during leukemic progression, the first one outgrows and the latter one disappears. Thus, the leukemic evolution of BPDCN could be driven by a major *TET2* mutated clone.

Szczepaniak and colleagues[24] recently published a work of targeted sequencing on 1 BPDCN patient. At diagnosis, the patient presented in both peripheral blood and bone marrow 2 nonsense mutations of *ASXL1* gene and 1 missense mutation of *TET2* gene. Apart from *TET2* and *ASXL1*, they identified a missense mutation in the neurofibromatosis-1 tumor suppressor gene, *NF1*, in the tumor DNA and also in the germline DNA. The presence of *NF1* germline mutation in a BPDCN patient *TET2* mutated led the authors to hypothesize a cooperative role of *NF1* in the promotion of cancer cell proliferation and tumor progression.

EPIGENETIC PATHWAY GENE MUTATIONS

Recent NGS-based discovery efforts in BPDCN have demonstrated that epigenetic factors were recurrently mutated, with about half of patients harboring at least 1 mutated epigenetic pathway gene.[12,17]

Functional enrichment analysis of the whole-exome mutational data, reported by Sapienza and colleagues,[17] showed that in BPDCN the epigenetic biological process was the most frequently affected by recurrent and deleterious mutations (frameshift, nonsense) predicted to disrupt functional protein integrity.

The most recurrently genes in BPDCN were 2 epigenetic modifiers: *ASXL1* and *TET2*.

ASXL1

ASXL1 is a component of the *PRC2* that mediates gene silencing through methylation of histone H3 lysine 27 (H3K27me3).[25] Recurrent *ASXL1* mutations are found in various hematologic malignancies and are associated with a poor prognosis.[26,27] Most *ASXL1* mutations encountered in myeloid disorders result in a deficiency of ASXL1 functionality.[28] To this regard, as demonstrated by in vitro and in vivo experiments, the depletion of *ASXL1* is able to promote myeloid transformation through impaired PRC2-mediated H3K27 methylation.[25] In BPDCN, most ASXL1 mutations are nonsense or frameshift and are located within or upstream of the catalytic domain of the proteins, potentially leading to its functional disruption.[29,30]

TET2

TET2 catalyzes the oxidation of 5-methylcytosine into 5-hydroxymethylcytosine to promote DNA demethylation.[31,32] Its genomic deletions or mutations are described prevalently in adult hematologic malignancies, including AML, MDS, and MPN.[32] *TET2* plays important roles in hematopoiesis, where it promotes the self-renewal of stem cells and lineage commitment and terminal differentiation of monocytes.[33] Its deletion is associated with DNA hypermethylation and abnormal gene expression in hematopoietic cells and is able to induce myeloid and lymphoid malignancies in mice.[34,35] In BPDCN, as described in other blood cancers, *TET2* mutations spread along all the exons and are often frameshift or nonsense, potentially damaging for the protein integrity.[17]

CLINICAL IMPACT OF EPIGENETIC MUTATIONS

In BPDCN, the clinical impact of the epigenetic modifier mutations has been evaluated by Menezes and colleagues,[12] who appreciated a significant reduction in the overall survival (OS) of patients mutated in any of the following DNA methylation genes: *TET2*, *IDH1/2*, *DNMT3A*, with respect to the unmutated ones (median 11 months vs 79 months; $P = .047$).

Thus, mutations of methylation genes may exert a negative prognostic value in BPDCN. However, these data need to be corroborated by a larger set of patients.

In myeloid malignancies, correlations between epigenetic gene mutations and prognosis have been debated; *TET2* mutations have a negative prognostic value in normal karyotype-AML,[36] whereas its effect on MDS[27] and MPN patients is less clear.[37] IDH1/2 mutations do not seem to exert any significant influence on the prognosis of MDS[26,27] and MPN patients,[37,38] whereas more univocally, *DNMT3A* mutations correlate with a shortened OS in patients with AML[39,40] or MDS.[41]

EPIGENETICS

The observation that genes encoding epigenetic regulators are among the most mutated factors in BPDCN strongly pointed to a role of epigenome dysregulation in its pathogenesis. In keeping with this, the integration of mutational data with other multi-omics information enlightened new critical epigenetic features of BPDCN.

Sapienza and colleagues[17] analyzed a set of BPDCN patients at gene expression and histone methylation/acetylation levels, which according to WES results, were mutated in various epigenetic pathway genes. The profile of trimethylation or acetylation signals on the histone H3 lysine 27 (H3K27me3/ac) allowed for the mapping of the genes transcriptionally turned on or turned off by epigenetic signals. BPDCN patients converged on the same pattern of H3K27 acetylation and, of relevance, a set of aberrantly overexpressed cell-cycle genes turned out to be acetylated in their promoters. Thus, in BPDCN, the abnormal tumor cell proliferation may be due to the alteration in the distribution of acetylation/methylation histone signals, specifically H3K27me3/ac.

As expected, the mutations of epigenetic pathway genes encountered in these patients induced a profound perturbation in the methylation program. Gene set enrichment analysis of RNA sequencing data presented a significant deregulation of 2 methylation gene signatures, driven by the KDM5B[34] histone-demethylase and PRMT5[35] methyltransferase-associated genes, respectively. Of note, BPDCN patients also exhibited a signature of genes responsive to decitabine, a DNA hypomethylating agent (HMA). In the light of this specific indication, useful for preclinical studies design, BPDCN mouse models engrafted with CAL-1 cell line were injected with different combinations of the following epigenetic drugs: azacitidine, decitabine, and romidepsin, with bortezomib and lenalidomide already known to be valid for BPDCN treatment.[42,43] The combined administration of HMAs, namely azacitidine and decitabine, was shown to be the most effective in tumor growth inhibition and offered new perspectives for phase 1 clinical trials.[17]

Emadali and colleagues[16] identified a group of BPDCN patients with deletion of the glucocorticoid resistance gene, namely N3RC1. Of note, these patients followed a more aggressive clinical behavior with respect to the undeleted ones. In vitro experiments on the BPDCN CAL-1 cell line demonstrated that N3RC1 silencing correlated with attenuation of glucocorticoid receptor signaling; acquisition of glucocorticoid resistance as in primary samples; enrichment of EZH2-loss-of-function gene signatures; global reduction of H3K27me3 level; and upregulation of PRC2 target genes, overall the HOXA genes. In other words, the N3RC1 loss may affect EZH2 functionality and alter the correct epigenetic signaling, with consequent derepression of otherwise silenced genes.

More detailed structural analysis of N3RC1 locus revealed, in 1 patient, the gene fusion of NR3C1 to a long-noncoding RNA, namely lincRNA-3q. LincRNA-3q was discovered to be consistently overexpressed among all the BPDCN patients whereby cell-cycle progression may be promoted through the activation of E2F-target genes, as suggested by in vitro experiments on the CAL-1 cell line. In CAL-1 cancer cells, Emadali and colleagues[16] also discovered that lincRNA-3q promoter was irregularly bound by a bromodomain and extraterminal (BET) domain protein, called BRD4, an epigenetic reader that stimulates gene transcription, and more specifically, messenger RNA elongation. Of clinical relevance, in many cancer types, BRD4 and BET proteins more generally, it can be successfully shut down by BET inhibitors (BETi).[44,45] Thus, Emadali and colleagues developed a BPDCN mouse model for testing the efficacy of BETi. As expected, BETi reversed the abnormal lincRNA-3q overexpression and arrested the BPDCN proliferation, adding a novel as well as encouraging option for BPDCN therapeutic strategy.

Glucocorticoid receptor signaling was recognized as a modulator of the BPDCN epigenetic program; its deficiency, because of NR3C1 deletion, may be linked to the reduction in the repressive signal H3K27me3-PRC2–mediated and to the irregular binding of BRD4 to the lncRNA-3q. In turn, the lnc-RNA-3q overexpression would engage further rounds of epigenetic reprogramming leading to the misregulation of E2F activity and the activation of leukemia stem cell programs. For the first time, the critical role of long-noncoding RNA in BPDCN tumorigenesis was evidenced, and an innovative treatment option based on the use of BET inhibitors was suggested.

To identify BPDCN molecular dependencies, Ceribelli and colleagues[46] performed a loss-of-function RNA interference (RNAi) screen in the CAL-1 BPDCN cell line and identified TCF4 as a master transcriptional regulator that sustains BPDCN malignancy. TCF4 overexpression was validated in a larger cohort of patients and became a new diagnostic BPDCN marker. Apart from TCF4, RNAi analysis identified a central role for the epigenetic reader, BRD4. Then, to find new therapeutic strategy, a small molecule drug screen was performed that, according to RNAi finding relative to BRD4, indicated the BETi as a promising effective treatment. RNA sequencing of in vitro and in vivo BPDCN models, before and after administration of BETi or *TCF4* silencing, revealed that the transcriptional changes after the 2 treatments were largely overlapping. In multiple cancer types, the successful cytotoxic activity of BETi was ascribed to the targeting of key oncogenes, dependent on superenhancers (SEs), regulatory domains highly enriched in BRD4 binding proteins.[47] Thus, to understand the mechanism of action of BETi in BPDCN, a BRD4-ChIP sequencing of CAL-1 cell line was performed. Ceribelli and colleagues built the first BRD4-SE map of BPDCN and identified *TCF4* as a top ranked gene, highly interconnected to BRD4-SE regions, targeted by BETi, as shown by in vivo BPDCN mouse models.

In conclusion, it was clearly shown that BPDCN survival relied on a TCF4-centered transcriptional network, epigenetically regulated by BRD4 proteins and successfully knocked down by BETi.

SUMMARY

It is now well documented that BPDCN has epigenetic modifier genes recurrently mutated and transcriptional methylation signatures aberrantly overexpressed, strongly accentuating the role of epigenome dysregulation in BPDCN pathogenesis. BPDCN displays a transcriptional profile well responsive to HMAs and a cell survival strictly dependent on the bromodomain protein BRD4, effectively knocked down by BETi.

Thus, therapeutic targeting of the epigenome turned out to be an attractive strategy for the BPDCN cure: the HMAs azacitidine and decitabine have raised great interest as an innovative treatment approach, alone and in combination with other novel agents.[17,48,49] Venetoclax, a selective BCL2 inhibitor,[50] in combination with HMAs, has induced a significant clinical response in relapsed/refractory patients,[51] and Tagraxofusp (SL-401), a CD123-targeted therapy, successfully producing disease remission,[52] may be ineffective in some refractory BPDCN patients, but treatment with azacitidine could restore Tagraxofusp sensitivity.[53]

Targeted epigenetic therapies are at the early stages of development, but the prospects are exciting. However, before epigenetic therapies can become the pillar of the BPDCN cure, more preclinical studies are needed in order to define the molecular consequences of the single epigenetic gene mutation, to predict the epigenetic drug efficacy, and, finally, to match each patient with the most appropriate targeted epigenetic-based therapy.

DISCLOSURE

The authors have nothing to disclose.

REFERENCES

1. WHO classification of tumours of haematopoietic and lymphoid tissues. In: Swerdlow SH, Campo E, Harris NL, et al, editors. World Health Organization classification of tumours. 4th edition. Lyon (France): International Agency for Research on Cancer; 2017. p. 173–8.

2. Khoury JD, Medeiros LJ, Manning JT, et al. CD56(+) TdT(+) blastic natural killer cell tumor of the skin: a primitive systemic malignancy related to myelomonocytic leukemia. Cancer 2002;94(9):2401–8.

3. Petrella T, Comeau MR, Maynadié M, et al. "Agranular CD4+ CD56+ hematodermic neoplasm" (blastic NK-cell lymphoma) originates from a population of CD56+ precursor cells related to plasmacytoid monocytes. Am J Surg Pathol 2002;26(7):852–62.

4. Lúcio P, Parreira A, Orfao A. CD123hi dendritic cell lymphoma: an unusual case of non-Hodgkin lymphoma. Ann Intern Med 1999;131(7):549–50.

5. Chaperot L, Bendriss N, Manches O, et al. Identification of a leukemic counterpart of the plasmacytoid dendritic cells. Blood 2001;97(10):3210–7.

6. Mullighan CG. TET2 mutations in myelodysplasia and myeloid malignancies. Nat Genet 2009;41(7):766–7.

7. Jardin F, Ruminy P, Parmentier F, et al. TET2 and TP53 mutations are frequently observed in blastic plasmacytoid dendritic cell neoplasm. Br J Haematol 2011; 153(3):413–6.

8. Alayed K, Patel KP, Konoplev S, et al. TET2 mutations, myelodysplastic features, and a distinct immunoprofile characterize blastic plasmacytoid dendritic cell neoplasm in the bone marrow. Am J Hematol 2013;88(12):1055–61.

9. Taylor J, Kim SS, Stevenson KE, et al. Loss-of-function mutations in the splicing factor ZRSR2 are common in blastic plasmacytoid dendritic cell neoplasm and have male predominance. Blood 2013;122:741.

10. Sichien D, Scott CL, Martens L, et al. IRF8 transcription factor controls survival and function of terminally differentiated conventional and plasmacytoid dendritic cells, respectively. Immunity 2016;45(3):626–40.

11. Togami K, Madan V, Li J, et al. Blastic plasmacytoid dendritic cell neoplasm (BPDCN) harbors frequent splicesosome mutations that cause aberrant RNA splicing affecting genes critical in pDC differentiation and function. Blood 2016; 128(22):738.

12. Menezes J, Acquadro F, Wiseman M, et al. Exome sequencing reveals novel and recurrent mutations with clinical impact in blastic plasmacytoid dendritic cell neoplasm. Leukemia 2014;28(4):823–9.

13. Cytlak U, Resteu A, Bogaert D, et al. Ikaros family zinc finger 1 regulates dendritic cell development and function in humans. Nat Commun 2018;9(1):1239.

14. Stenzinger A, Endris V, Pfarr N, et al. Targeted ultra-deep sequencing reveals recurrent and mutually exclusive mutations of cancer genes in blastic plasmacytoid dendritic cell neoplasm. Oncotarget 2014;5(15):6404–13.

15. Tsagarakis NJ, Kentrou NA, Papadimitriou KA, et al. Acute lymphoplasmacytoid dendritic cell (DC2) leukemia: results from the Hellenic Dendritic Cell Leukemia Study Group. Leuk Res 2010;34(4):438–46.

16. Emadali A, Hoghoughi N, Duley S, et al. Haploinsufficiency for NR3C1, the gene encoding the glucocorticoid receptor, in blastic plasmacytoid dendritic cell neoplasms. Blood 2016;127(24):3040–53.

17. Sapienza MR, Abate F, Melle F, et al. Blastic plasmacytoid dendritic cell neoplasm: genomics mark epigenetic dysregulation as a primary therapeutic target. Haematologica 2019;104(4):729–37.

18. Lee K-H, Park J-W, Sung H-S, et al. PHF2 histone demethylase acts as a tumor suppressor in association with p53 in cancer. Oncogene 2015;34(22):2897–909.

19. Subtil-Rodríguez A, Vázquez-Chávez E, Ceballos-Chávez M, et al. The chromatin remodeler CHD8 is required for E2F-dependent transcription activation of S-phase genes. Nucleic Acids Res 2014;42(4):2185–96.

20. Guarini A, Marinelli M, Tavolaro S, et al. ATM gene alterations in chronic lymphocytic leukemia patients induce a distinct gene expression profile and predict disease progression. Haematologica 2012;97(1):47–55.

21. Simon M, Grandage VL, Linch DC, et al. Constitutive activation of the Wnt/beta-catenin signalling pathway in acute myeloid leukaemia. Oncogene 2005;24(14): 2410–20.

22. Kuo Y-H, Zaidi SK, Gornostaeva S, et al. Runx2 induces acute myeloid leukemia in cooperation with Cbfbeta-SMMHC in mice. Blood 2009;113(14):3323–32.

23. Ladikou E, Ottolini B, Nawaz N, et al. Clonal evolution in the transition from cutaneous disease to acute leukemia suggested by liquid biopsy in blastic plasmacytoid dendritic cell neoplasm. Haematologica 2018;103(5):e196–9.

24. Szczepaniak A, Machnicki M, Gniot M, et al. Germline missense NF1 mutation in an elderly patient with a blastic plasmacytoid dendritic cell neoplasm. Int J Hematol 2019;110(1):102–6.

25. Abdel-Wahab O, Adli M, LaFave LM, et al. ASXL1 mutations promote myeloid transformation through loss of PRC2-mediated gene repression. Cancer Cell 2012;22(2):180–93.

26. Abdel-Wahab O, Pardanani A, Patel J, et al. Concomitant analysis of EZH2 and ASXL1 mutations in myelofibrosis, chronic myelomonocytic leukemia and blast-phase myeloproliferative neoplasms. Leukemia 2011;25(7):1200–2.

27. Bejar R, Stevenson K, Abdel-Wahab O, et al. Clinical effect of point mutations in myelodysplastic syndromes. N Engl J Med 2011;364(26):2496–506.

28. Balasubramani A, Larjo A, Bassein JA, et al. Cancer-associated ASXL1 mutations may act as gain-of-function mutations of the ASXL1-BAP1 complex. Nat Commun 2015;6(1):7307.

29. Yannakou CK, Jones K, McBean M, et al. ASXL1 c.1934dup;p.Gly646Trpfs*12—a true somatic alteration requiring a new approach. Blood Cancer J 2017; 7(12):656.

30. Delhommeau F, Dupont S, Valle VD, et al. Mutation in TET2 in myeloid cancers. N Engl J Med 2009;360(22):2289–301.

31. Cai Z, Kotzin JJ, Ramdas B, et al. Inhibition of inflammatory signaling in Tet2 mutant preleukemic cells mitigates stress-induced abnormalities and clonal hematopoiesis. Cell Stem Cell 2018;23(6):833–49.e5.

32. Feng Y, Li X, Cassady K, et al. TET2 function in hematopoietic malignancies, immune regulation, and DNA repair. Front Oncol 2019;9:210.

33. Solary E, Bernard OA, Tefferi A, et al. The ten-eleven translocation-2 (TET2) gene in hematopoiesis and hematopoietic diseases. Leukemia 2014;28(3):485–96.

34. Li Z, Cai X, Cai C-L, et al. Deletion of Tet2 in mice leads to dysregulated hematopoietic stem cells and subsequent development of myeloid malignancies. Blood 2011;118(17):4509–18.

35. Rasmussen KD, Jia G, Johansen JV, et al. Loss of TET2 in hematopoietic cells leads to DNA hypermethylation of active enhancers and induction of leukemogenesis. Genes Dev 2015;29(9):910–22.

36. Metzeler KH, Maharry K, Radmacher MD, et al. TET2 mutations improve the new European LeukemiaNet risk classification of acute myeloid leukemia: a Cancer and Leukemia Group B study. J Clin Oncol 2011;29(10):1373–81.

37. Tefferi A, Pardanani A, Lim K-H, et al. TET2 mutations and their clinical correlates in polycythemia vera, essential thrombocythemia and myelofibrosis. Leukemia 2009;23(5):905–11.

38. Tefferi A, Jimma T, Sulai NH, et al. IDH mutations in primary myelofibrosis predict leukemic transformation and shortened survival: clinical evidence for leukemogenic collaboration with JAK2V617F. Leukemia 2012;26(3):475–80.

39. Ley TJ, Ding L, Walter MJ, et al. DNMT3A mutations in acute myeloid leukemia. N Engl J Med 2010;363(25):2424–33.

40. Yan X-J, Xu J, Gu Z-H, et al. Exome sequencing identifies somatic mutations of DNA methyltransferase gene DNMT3A in acute monocytic leukemia. Nat Genet 2011;43(4):309–15.
41. Walter MJ, Ding L, Shen D, et al. Recurrent DNMT3A mutations in patients with myelodysplastic syndromes. Leukemia 2011;25(7):1153–8.
42. for the AIRC 5xMille consortium 'Genetics-driven targeted management of lymphoid malignancies' and the Italian Registry on Blastic Plasmacytoid Dendritic Cell Neoplasm, Sapienza MR, Fuligni F, Agostinelli C, et al. Molecular profiling of blastic plasmacytoid dendritic cell neoplasm reveals a unique pattern and suggests selective sensitivity to NF-kB pathway inhibition. Leukemia 2014; 28(8):1606–16.
43. Agliano A, Martin-Padura I, Marighetti P, et al. Therapeutic effect of lenalidomide in a novel xenograft mouse model of human blastic NK cell lymphoma/blastic plasmacytoid dendritic cell neoplasm. Clin Cancer Res 2011;17(19):6163–73.
44. Shin HY. Targeting super-enhancers for disease treatment and diagnosis. Mol Cell 2018;41(6):506–14.
45. Jang MK, Mochizuki K, Zhou M, et al. The bromodomain protein Brd4 is a positive regulatory component of P-TEFb and stimulates RNA polymerase II-dependent transcription. Mol Cell 2005;19(4):523–34.
46. Ceribelli M, Hou ZE, Kelly PN, et al. A druggable TCF4- and BRD4-dependent transcriptional network sustains malignancy in blastic plasmacytoid dendritic cell neoplasm. Cancer Cell 2016;30(5):764–78.
47. Lovén J, Hoke HA, Lin CY, et al. Selective inhibition of tumor oncogenes by disruption of super-enhancers. Cell 2013;153(2):320–34.
48. Laribi K, Denizon N, Ghnaya H, et al. Blastic plasmacytoid dendritic cell neoplasm: the first report of two cases treated by 5-azacytidine. Eur J Haematol 2014;93(1):81–5.
49. Khwaja R, Daly A, Wong M, et al. Azacitidine in the treatment of blastic plasmacytoid dendritic cell neoplasm: a report of 3 cases. Leuk Lymphoma 2016;57(11): 2720–2.
50. Montero J, Stephansky J, Cai T, et al. Blastic plasmacytoid dendritic cell neoplasm is dependent on BCL2 and sensitive to venetoclax. Cancer Discov 2017;7(2):156–64.
51. DiNardo CD, Rausch CR, Benton C, et al. Clinical experience with the BCL2-inhibitor venetoclax in combination therapy for relapsed and refractory acute myeloid leukemia and related myeloid malignancies. Am J Hematol 2018;93(3): 401–7.
52. Pemmaraju N, Lane AA, Sweet KL, et al. Tagraxofusp in blastic plasmacytoid dendritic-cell neoplasm. N Engl J Med 2019;380(17):1628–37.
53. Togami K, Pastika T, Stephansky J, et al. DNA methyltransferase inhibition overcomes diphthamide pathway deficiencies underlying CD123-targeted treatment resistance. J Clin Invest 2019;129(11):5005–19.

Cytogenetics of Blastic Plasmacytoid Dendritic Cell Neoplasm
Chromosomal Rearrangements and DNA Copy-Number Alterations

Kana Sakamoto, MD, PhD[a,b], Kengo Takeuchi, MD, PhD[a,b,c],*

KEYWORDS

- BPDCN • Chromosomal aberration • Tumor suppressor gene • Translocation
- MYC • MYB • t(6;8) (p21;q24) • Immunoblastoid

KEY POINTS

- Approximately 60% of cases of BPDCN show complex karyotypes and losses are more frequently found than copy-number gains.
- Multiple losses of tumor suppressor genes, especially those regulating the G1/S cell-cycle transition (eg, CDKN2A, CDKN2B, CDKN1B, and RB1), are found in BPDCN and possibly contribute to its pathogenesis.
- 8q24 rearrangement, most frequently with 6p21 harboring RUNX2, is found in one-third of cases of BPDCN and is associated with immunoblastoid cytomorphology and MYC expression.
- MYB rearrangement is detected in 20% of BPDCN patients, especially in children and young adults. The rearrangement induces the truncation of the negative regulator domain of MYB.

INTRODUCTION

Blastic plasmacytoid dendritic cell neoplasm (BPDCN) is a rare, skin-tropic hematopoietic malignancy. It is derived from the precursors of plasmacytoid dendritic cells (pDCs) and the tumor cells of BPDCN express pDC markers (eg, CD123, CD303/

Funding: This work was supported in part by grants from AMED (to K. Sakamoto), JSPS KAKENHI (to K. Sakamoto), and the Uehara Memorial Foundation (to K. Sakamoto).
[a] Pathology Project for Molecular Targets, The Cancer Institute, Japanese Foundation for Cancer Research, 3-8-31 Ariake, Koto, Tokyo 135-8550, Japan; [b] Division of Pathology, The Cancer Institute, Japanese Foundation for Cancer Research, Tokyo, Japan; [c] Clinical Pathology Center, The Cancer Institute Hospital, Japanese Foundation for Cancer Research, Tokyo, Japan
* Corresponding author.
E-mail address: kentakeuchi-tky@umin.net

Hematol Oncol Clin N Am 34 (2020) 523–538
https://doi.org/10.1016/j.hoc.2020.01.003
0889-8588/20/© 2020 Elsevier Inc. All rights reserved.

hemonc.theclinics.com

BDCA2, TCL1, TCF4, BCL11A, and CD2AP). Before the recognition of the relevance to pDCs, this disease used to be called by various names, such as "agranular CD4[+]CD56[+] haematodermic neoplasm" and "blastic NK-cell lymphoma."[1] The differential diagnosis includes acute myeloid leukemia (AML); the precise diagnosis is difficult without careful evaluation of the pDC-specific markers in combination.[2]

Most cases of BPDCN with analyzable karyotyping results show complex karyotypes (57%–66%).[1,3] The pattern is heterogeneous with some recurrently altered, mostly deleted, regions. Through analysis using conventional karyotyping and comparative genomic hybridization (CGH), no specific chromosomal abnormalities had been demonstrated in BPDCN. However, recurrent genomic rearrangements involving the *MYB* family genes and *MYC* were found in subsets of BPDCN in 2017 and 2018,[4–6] whereas translocations involving these genes are rarely reported in myeloid malignancies.[7] The scope of this paper is to review copy-number alterations and rearrangements demonstrated in BPDCN in detail.

Copy-Number Alteration

The results of conventional karyotyping in cases of BPDCN have been shown in various case reports and small case series.[8–10] The first report of cytogenetic investigation in BPDCN with a substantial number of cases was by Leroux[11] in 2002. He analyzed 21 cases of CD4+ CD56+ dendritic cell (DC2) acute leukemia using conventional and fluorescence in situ hybridization (FISH)/24-color karyotyping. Clonal, mostly complex chromosome aberrations were detected in 66% of patients (14/21 cases). They found gross genomic imbalances with a predominance of losses over gains. Six major recurrent chromosomal targets were identified: 5q (72%), 12p (64%), 13q (64%), 6q (50%), 15q (43%), and 9 (28%, usually monosomy 9), although no single anomaly specific to this disease was found. In 2016, Tang and colleagues[12] conducted a literature review of 46 cases of BPDCN with abnormal karyotypes. They found the same 6 major chromosomal aberrations identified by Leroux with a deviant frequency for each chromosome. Of note, some of the cases included were not evaluated for pDC-specific markers, and thus other diagnoses could be given if analyzed thoroughly.

In the early 2000s, CGH began to be used in studies of BPDCN.[13–16] The introduction of the high-resolution array-based CGH (aCGH) in the late 2000s enabled the detailed analysis of regions with recurrent abnormalities. In 2007, Dijkman and colleagues[17] first reported an integrated analysis of gene expression profiling and aCGH in BPDCN. In this study, the skin samples of patients with BPDCN (N = 5) and cutaneous AML (N = 6) were examined. The authors tried to elucidate the genetic features of BPDCN in comparison with cutaneous AML because these 2 conditions showed similar clinical and immunophenotypical behavior, making the differential diagnosis difficult. They showed distinct patterns of chromosomal aberrations in these 2 conditions. As shown in the studies using low-resolution analysis, losses were more frequently found than low copy-number gains in BPDCN, characterized by recurrent deletion of 4q34, chromosome 9 (9p13-p11 and 9q12-q34, including cases with monosomy 9), and 13q12-q31. The 21 genes located in 13q12.11-13q31.1 with decreased expression (compared with the cutaneous AML cases) included the tumor suppressor genes (TSGs): *RB1*, *LATS2*, and *KPNA3*. The subsequent 3 studies using aCGH with higher resolution performed around 2010 (by Jardin and colleagues,[18] Wiesner and colleagues,[19] and Lucioni and colleagues[20]) revealed multiple losses of TSGs, especially the genes controlling the G1/S cell-cycle transition (eg, *CDKN2A*, *CDKN2B*, *CDKN1B*, and *RB1*) in BPDCN. Of the total of 44 cases analyzed, the most frequently deleted regions were chromosome 9 or 9p (27/44, 61%), 12p13

(26/44, 59%), and 13q (24/44, 55%). The coexistence of these chromosomal aberrations leading to a combination of deletions of several TSGs, which was infrequent in lymphoid and myeloid tumors, was shown to be a peculiar genomic feature of BPDCN.[11,17,18,20,21] The candidate genes located in the recurrently deleted regions, which are relatively well studied, are reviewed in the following sections and **Table 1**.

Chromosome 9

9p21.3 harbors CDKN2A and CDKN2B, encoding the cell-cycle inhibitors $p16^{INK4a}$ and $p15^{INK4b}$, respectively. These proteins arrest the cell cycle by inhibiting the CDK4/6-mediated phosphorylation of RB1.[22] Wiesner and colleagues[19] found the loss of 9p21.3 in 7 of 14 cases of BPDCN (1 biallelic, 6 monoallelic). In immunohistochemistry (IHC), all 14 cases were negative for $p16^{INK4a}$, suggesting a complete loss of function of the protein. This indicated that other mechanisms, such as mutations or epigenetic modifications, were occurring in the undeleted alleles. Lucioni and colleagues[20] identified the deletion of the 9p21.3 locus in 14 of 21 cases of BPDCN (67%, 5 homozygous, 9 heterozygous) by aCGH and FISH. Although IHC for $p16^{INK4a}$ was negative in all samples, the survival probability was lower in the patients with biallelic loss of 9p21.3 (11 months for biallelic loss, 26 months for heterozygous loss). The deletion of CDKN2A was demonstrated in the studies using next-generation sequencing. Stenzinger and colleagues[23] performed a targeted sequencing of 33 cases of BPDCN and found that CDKN2A was the most frequently deleted gene among 50 commonly mutated cancer genes (9/33 cases, 27%), followed by RB1 (3/33, 9%), PTEN (1/33, 3%), and TP53 (1/33, 3%). Sapienza and colleagues[24] detected the deletion of CDKN2A in 8/14 (57%) cases of BPDCN using whole exome sequencing.

Chromosome 12

12p13 harbors CDKN1B, encoding the cell-cycle inhibitor $p27^{KIP1}$, which is a dose-dependent haploinsufficient tumor suppressor; the decreased expression of the protein was shown to drive the cell cycle by stabilizing cyclin D-dependent kinases.[19,25,26] Wiesner and colleagues[19] reported loss of 12p13 as the most frequent finding in the aCGH analysis of BPDCN (8/14 cases, 64%). They also performed IHC for $p27^{KIP1}$ and found weak nuclear expression in the tumor cells of 13/14 cases, confirming the monoallelic loss of CDKN1B.

12p13 also contains ETV6, a gene encoding a transcriptional repressor that plays a critical role in hematopoiesis and embryonic development.[27] Translocations, numerical aberrations, and mutations have been reported in many hematologic malignancies. Tang and colleagues[12] reported a BPDCN case with complicated chromosomal abnormalities involving chromosomes 12 and 22 that resulted in a simultaneous partial deletion of ETV6 and EWSR1 (22q12). The same group later reported a high prevalence of monoallelic and biallelic loss of 12p/ETV6 in BPDCN using karyotyping (8/30 cases, 27%) and FISH (9/13 cases, 69%) in 2018.[3] Of note, ETV6 FISH could detect 12p/ETV6 deletion in the specimens that showed normal karyotypes and those in which no BPDCN involvement was detected with IHC.

Chromosome 13

13q contains RB1 (13q14) and LATS2 (13q12), both of which are TSGs. Patnaik and colleagues[28] performed whole-exome sequencing using chronic myelomonocytic leukemia (CMML) and transformed BPDCN samples from the same patient. Biallelic loss of RB1 (a truncating mutation along with loss of heterozygosity) was detected only in the BPDCN sample, suggesting its contribution to a BPDCN phenotypic transformation of CMML.

Table 1
Commonly altered chromosomal regions and the candidate genes in BPDCN

Reference	Samples (N)	Methods	Abnormality	Chromosomal Regions	Candidate Genes	Positive/Evaluated (%)
Leroux,[11] 2002	BM (17), PB (3), LN (1)	R-banding, FISH	Deletion/translocation	5q		10/14 (72) [10/20 (50)][a]
			Deletion/translocations	12p (12p13)		9/14 (64) [9/20 (45)][a]
			Deletion	13q (13q13–21)		9/14 (64) [9/20 (45)][a]
			Deletion/translocation	6q (6q23–qter)		7/14 (50) [7/20 (35)][a]
			Deletion/inversion	15q		6/14 (43) [6/20 (30)][a]
			Deletion	Chromosome 9	CDKN2A	4/14 (28) [4/20 (20)][a]
Dijkman et al,[17] 2007	Skin	aCGH, microarray	Deletion	9q12–q34.3	CDC14B, DBC1, SYK	5/5 (100)
			Deletion	13q12.11–q31.1	KPNA3, LATS2, RB1	4/5 (80)
			Deletion	9p13.2–p11.2		4/5 (80)
			Deletion	4q34.1–q34.2		4/5 (80)
Jardin et al,[18] 2009	PB (5), BM (3), LN (1)	aCGH, PCR	Deletion	Chromosome 9 (9p)	CDKN2A/CDKN2B	6/9 (67)
			Deletion	13q13.3–q14.2	RB1	7/9 (78)
			Deletion	12p13.2	CDKN1B, ETV6	6/9 (67)
			Deletion	17p	TP53	3/9 (33)
			Deletion	5q	MSH3, miRNA coding genes, SMAD5, MCC, APC	4/9 (44)

Study	Source	Method	Type	Cytoband	Gene	Frequency
Wiesner et al,[19] 2010	Skin	aCGH, IHC	Deletion	12p13.2	CDKN1B, ETV6	8/14 (64)
			Deletion	9p21.3	CDKN2A, CDKN2B, ARF	7/14 (50)
			Deletion	9q34		7/14 (50)
			Deletion	13q12.11-q34	RB1	6/14 (43)
			Deletion	15q11.2-q26.3		5/14 (36)
			Deletion	19p13.3-p13.4		4/14 (29)
			Deletion	3p22.2-p21.1	PTPN23	4/14 (29)
			Deletion	5q32-q35.2		3/14 (21)
			Deletion	6q23.3-q27	PARK2	3/14 (21)
			Deletion	7p22.3-p22.1	MAD1L1	3/14 (21)
			Deletion	21q22.3		3/14 (21)
Lucioni et al,[20] 2011	NA	aCGH, FISH, IHC	Deletion	9p21.3	CDKN2A/CDKN2B, MTAP	14/21 (67)
			Deletion	13q13.1-q14.3	RB1, CCNA1, KPNAP3, hsa-mir-320d-1, hsa-mir-621, hsa-mir-16-1, hsa-mir-15a.	11/21 (52)
			Deletion	13q11-q12	LATS2	11/21 (52)
			Deletion	12p13.2-p13.1	CDKN1B	12/21 (57)
			Deletion	7p12.2	IKZF1	4/21 (19)
Petrella et al,[15] 2012	Skin, BM	aCGH, FISH	Deletion	6q11.1-q16.3		1/1
			Deletion	12p12.1-p13.31	ETV6	1/1
			Deletion	13q13.1-q13.3		1/1
			Deletion	13q14.11-q14.12		1/1
			Deletion	13q21.1-q21.31		1/1
	BM		Deletion	2p11.2		1/1
			Deletion	2p16.1		1/1
			Deletion	2p21-p22.1		1/1
			Deletion	2p24.1		1/1
			Deletion	5q23.2		1/1
			Deletion	5q31.3-q33.1		1/1
			Deletion	5q33.2-q33.3		1/1

(continued on next page)

Table 1
(continued)

Reference	Samples (N)	Methods	Abnormality	Chromosomal Regions	Candidate Genes	Positive/Evaluated (%)
Oiso et al,[16] 2012	Skin	aCGH	Deletion	1p31.3–33	CDKN2Clp18, GADD45A, JUN, JAK1	1/1
			Deletion	9p/q	CDKN2A, CDKN2B, ARF	1/1
			Deletion	12p13.1–13.2	CDKN1B	1/1
			Deletion	13p/q	RB1	1/1
			Gain	16p/q (gain)		1/1
Fu et al,[31] 2013	BM	aCGH	Deletion	5q14.3–q31.3	HINT1(5q23.3)	1/1
Stenzinger et al,[23] 2014	Skin (32), nasopharynx (1)	Targeted sequencing	Deletion		CDKN2A	9/33 (27)
			Deletion		RB1	3/33 (9)
			Deletion		PTEN	1/33 (3)
			Deletion		TP53	1/33 (3)
Emadali et al,[32] 2016	Karyotyping: PB (11), BM (28), LN (1), NA (7)	R-banding, FISH, aCGH, targeted sequencing, microarray, ChIP sequencing	Deletion/ translocation	5q31	NR3C1	5q: 17/47 (38) NR3C1: 13/47 (28)
Tang et al,[12] 2016	BM, LN	G-banding, FISH, literature review	Translocation/ deletion	t(12;22) (p13;q12)	ETV6, EWSR1	1/1
Tang et al,[3] 2018	BM, skin	G-banding, aCGH (N = 2), FISH	Deletion/ translocation	12p13	ETV6	Conventional: 8/30 (27), FISH (BM): 9/13 (69)
Sapienza et al,[24] 2019	Skin	Whole exome sequencing	Deletion		CDKN2A	8/14 (57)

Abbreviations: aCGH, array-based CGH; BM, bone marrow; ChIP, chromatin immunoprecipitation; FISH, fluorescence in situ hybridization; IHC, immunohistochemistry; LN, lymph ncde; PB, peripheral blood.
[a] The number of the evaluated cases was 20 when the 6 cases with normal karyotype were included in the calculation.

Chromosome 17

In the study by Jardin and colleagues[18] performed in 2009, 3 of 9 cases of BPDCN (33%) harbored a partial or complete loss of 17p, and the commonly deleted region contained the *TP53* gene (17p13.1). No homozygous deletion of this gene was observed. Missense mutations were detected in 2 of the 3 cases, indicating a complete loss of p53 function. The mutations of *TP53* have been reported in BPDCN with various positive rates.[21,23,24,29,30]

Chromosome 5

Deletion of 5q is commonly found in myelodysplastic syndrome and AML, and 5q is known to contain multiple TSGs important in the pathogenesis of myeloid tumors.[1] Jardin and colleagues[18] found deletions in 5q in 3 of 9 cases of BPDCN and suggested *MSH3* (5q14.1), *SMAD5* (5q31.1), *MCC* (5q22.2), *APC* (5q22.2), and the micro RNA genes as candidate genes. Through combined analysis of their own case and the 3 cases with 5q alteration in the study of Jardin and colleagues,[18] Fu and colleagues[31] reported that the breakpoints on 5q in BPDCN could be heterogeneous and suggested *HINT1*, a TSG, as a candidate gene on 5q. In 2016, Emadali and colleagues[32] reported monoallelic deletion of *NR3C1*, a gene located in 5q31, which encodes the glucocorticoid receptor, in 13 of 47 cases of BPDCN (28%). Haploinsufficiency for *NR3C1* was associated with poor overall survival. They found the association between *NR3C1* deletion and the loss of EZH2 function using gene expression profiling, which suggested the role of *NR3C1* as a tumor suppressor. In a case with t(3;5)(q21;q31), *NR3C1* was fused to a long noncoding RNA gene at 3q21 (*lincRNA-3q*). The overexpression of lincRNA-3q was detected in a subset of BPDCN patients compared with normal pDCs. The knockdown of *lincRNA-3q* with shRNA impaired the cell growth of a BPDCN cell line (CAL-1) in xenografts. They also showed that bromodomain and extraterminal domain (BET) inhibition abrogated lincRNA-3q overexpression and the growth of the tumor in the xenograft model.

Chromosome 7

7p12.2 encompasses *IKZF1* (IKAROS family zinc finger 1) and was found to be deleted in 19% of cases of BPDCN in the study by Lucioni and colleagues.[20] The recurrent mutations of the IKAROS family genes (*IKZF1*, *IKZF2*, and *IKZF3*) were reported in 5/25 (20%) of patients with BPDCN by targeted sequencing in the study by Menezes and colleagues[30] in 2014. IKAROS, encoded by *IKZF1*, is a hematopoietic transcription factor that has crucial roles in lymphocyte development.[33,34] The mutations and deletions of *IKZF1* occur frequently in leukemias, such as B-lymphoblastic leukemia with *BCR-ABL1*.[35] Interestingly, the heterozygous mutation of *IKZF1* has been shown to reduce the number of pDCs and there has been accumulating evidence that shows the regulatory role of *IKZF1* in dendritic cell development.[34,36]

MYC Rearrangement

MYC, located at 8q24.21, is a well-known oncogene that has a wide range of functions in cell proliferation, growth, metabolism, and genome stability.[37] 8q24 rearrangement is found in Burkitt lymphoma, multiple myeloma, and other aggressive B cell lymphomas. In myeloid tumors, 8q24 rearrangement has been rarely reported,[38] except for t(3;8)(q26;q24) related to *MECOM* (*MDS1* and *EVI1* complex locus), located at 3q26.2, and *MYC/PVT1* at 8q24.[39]

There were sporadic reports of cases of BPDCN with 8q24 rearrangment,[31,40–44] but the positive rate, and the biological and clinical features were unclear. In 2018, we examined 118 cases of BPDCN and revealed the recurrent 8q24 rearrangement using *MYC* split FISH (41/109 cases, 38%). Interestingly, 8q24 rearrangement was strongly associated with "immunoblastoid" cytomorphology and MYC expression evaluated by IHC[5] (**Fig. 1**). MYC⁺BPDCN (both positive by FISH and IHC) and MYC⁻BPDCN (both negative) were clinically different in some aspects, including age and the skin lesion features. The response to therapies and the prognosis were shown to be worse in patients with MYC⁺BPDCN, although further examination is required due to the retrospective nature of the study. The immunophenotype was also different between cases of MYC⁺BPDCN and MYC⁻BPDCN. The positive rate for CD56 was significantly lower in MYC⁺BPDCN (78%, 32/41 cases) compared with cases of MYC⁻BPDCN (98%, 58/59 cases), and CD10 was more frequently positive in cases of MYC⁺BPDCN compared with cases of MYC⁻BPDCN (41% vs 6%). In functional analyses using BPDCN cell lines, CAL-1 (MYC⁺BPDCN) and PMDC05 (MYC⁻BPDCN), CAL-1 showed higher sensitivity to the inhibitors for BET and aurora kinases than PMDC05. These data suggested that MYC status could be a biomarker for potential therapeutic approaches for BPDCN using those inhibitors.

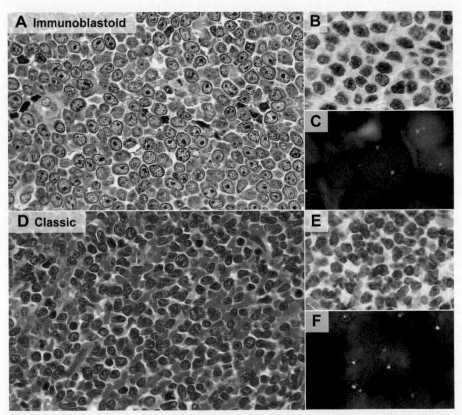

Fig. 1. The cytomorphology and MYC status in BPDCN. A representative MYC⁺BPDCN case showed (*A*) immunoblastoid cytomorphology (H&E) and (*B*) positivity for MYC immunostaining. (*A*) The immunoblastoid cells have a round-to-ovoid nucleus with a large centrally located nucleolus, resembling immunoblasts (activated B cells). (*C*) Split signals were observed via FISH for *MYC* in an immunoblastoid BPDCN case. A representative MYC⁻BPDCN case showed (*D*) classic cytomorphology (H&E). The classic neoplastic cells are medium-sized blast cells with irregular nuclei, fine chromatin, and one to several small nucleoli. (*E*) They were negative for MYC. (*F*) No split signals were observed via FISH for MYC in a classic BPDCN case.

The frequency of 8q24 rearrangement in BPDCN was reported as 12% (5/41 of cases of BPDCN) using conventional karyotyping in a case series.[6] The discrepancy in the positive rate between our data and the report indicates that conventional karyotyping is not enough to detect 8q24 rearrangement in BPDCN.

t(6;8)(p21;q24) was sporadically reported in BPDCN (**Table 2**).[6,11,31,32,40–43,45–47] In a case with the translocation, Nakamura and colleagues[43] identified a chimeric transcript of *SUPT3H* (6p21) and *PVT1* (50 kb downstream of *MYC*) in 2015. In our cohort, 56% of cases MYC$^+$BPDCN showed split signal patterns in *SUPT3H* split FISH, indicating that 6p21 is the most frequent partner locus in 8q24-rearranged cases of BPDCN. The genomic sequence of *SUPT3H* overlaps with *RUNX2*, a highly expressed[17] super-enhancer gene,[48] in BPDCN. Therefore, the translocation of super-enhancers close to or within *RUNX2* in the proximity of *MYC* was inferred as the mechanism of high expression of MYC in cases with t(6;8) (p21;q24)[5,31]; this was confirmed using CAL-1, a MYC$^+$BPDCN cell line harboring this translocation in 2019.[49] In a literature review of 16 BPDCN cases with *MYC* translocations, the cases with t(6;8)(p21;q24) (N = 11) were shown to have shorter median survival times.[45] In our MYC$^+$BPDCN cohort, there was no significant difference in overall survival between the cases with and without the *SUPT3H* split (unpublished data). The biological and clinical difference regarding the partner locus for 8q24 needs further evaluation.

Through the analysis from aCGH, Jardin and colleagues[18] reported that 2 of 9 BPDCN cases had deletion breakpoints close to *MYC*. In one of those cases, a 5.6-Mb deletion on 8q24 (8q24.21-q24.22), including the *PVT1* locus, moved *MYC* and miR-30b closer together and the expression of MYC was relatively high compared with other cases. The heterozygous loss of 8q24 (8q24.21-q24.22) was also detected using aCGH in 1 case by Lucioni and colleagues.[20] Interestingly, the tumor cells of the case shown in the picture seem to be immunoblastoid. MYC status was not examined for that case.

MYB Rearrangement

The *MYB* gene is located at 6q23.3 and encodes the MYB transcription factor. It is known to regulate cell-cycle progression and is implicated in many types of tumors, functioning as an oncogene.[50] One of the major mechanisms for MYB activation in cancer cells is the deletion or disruption of the regulatory C-terminal domains of MYB. This can be caused by alternative RNA splicing in leukemia and by rearrangements in several kinds of solid tumors, such as adenoid cystic carcinoma.[50] In BPDCN, Suzuki and colleagues[4] identified recurrent *MYB* rearrangements in 5 of 5 (100%) pediatric and 4 of 9 (44%) adult cases using RNA sequencing in 2017. The fusion genes included *MYB-PLEKHO1* (N = 3), *MYB-ZFAT* (N = 4), *MYB-DCPS* (N = 1), and *MYB-MIR3134* (N = 1). The products of these fusion genes retained the MYB transcriptional activation domain, whereas its negative regulator domain was truncated, indicating that these MYB derivatives were in active forms. Suzuki and colleagues confirmed the activation of MYB target genes on exogenous MYB-PLEKHO1 expression in 293T cells.

In our cohort, *MYB* rearrangement was detected in 19/96 (20%) BPDCN cases by split FISH assay.[5] In addition, we also identified a case with *MYBL1* rearrangement (1/95 cases, 1%).[5] *MYBL1* is located at 8q13.1 and the encoded protein has a similar structure with MYB; the recurrent *MYBL1* rearrangements have been reported in adenoid cystic carcinoma[51] and pediatric gliomas.[52] The median age of the patients with BPDCN with *MYB/MYBL1* rearrangements was 50 years (range 3–87 years), and 3 of 5 patients under 20 years old were included.[5] All examined cases of MYC$^+$BPDCN were negative for *MYB/MYBL1* rearrangement, whereas 18/51 (35%)

Table 2
Cases of blastic plasmacytoid dendritic cell neoplasm with t(6;8) (p21;q24) in the literature

Reference	Case No.	Other Reference	Age	Sex	Cytogenetics
Leroux,[11] 2002	24	Emadali et al,[32] 2016 (case 1), Chaperot,[46] 2001 (case GEN)	74	Male	49,XY,+add(6)(q21),-8,+2mar,+r[6]/49,idem,t(15;16)(?q21;?q21)[6]/49,idem,t(3;5)(?q21;?q31)[5] Ish wcp M-FISH 49,XY,+6,t(6;8)(p21;q24),+r(12),+20/49,idem,inv(15)(q1?4q2?3),t(16;16)(q?;q?)/49,idem,t(3;5)(q?21;q?31)[13]
Momoi et al,[40] 2002	1	Sakamoto et al,[5] 2018	69	Male	46,XY,add(5)(q11),add(5)(q31),t(6;8)(p21;q24),del(13)(q12q14),add(15)(q13)[9]
Maeda et al,[41] 2005	—	Emadali et al,[32] 2016 (case 2)	76	Male	45,X,-Y,+add(1)(q32),der(1;15)(q10;q10)[16]/45,X,-Y,+add(1)(q32),der(1;15)(q10;q10),t(6;8)(p21;q24),t(7;14)(q21;q11)[2]
Takiuchi et al,[42] 2012	—		74	Male	47,XY,t(6;8)(p21;q24),+r[20]
Fu et al,[31] 2013	—		67	Female	46,XX,del(5)(q13q33),t(6;8)(p21;q24)
Nakamura et al,[43] 2015	—	Sakamoto et al,[5] 2018	81	Male	Lymph node: 47,X,-Y t(6;8)(p21;q24),+add(7)(p11.2),+der(8)t(6;8),+20[17/20],46,XY [3/20] Bone marrow: 48,X,-Y,t(6;8)(p21;q24),+add(7)(p11.2),+der(8)t(6;8),+20 [5/13],49,idem,+mar1 t(6;8),+20 [2/13],49,idem,der(8)t(6;8),?t(9;15)(p22;q15),+mar1[2/13],46,XY[3/13]

Study	No.	Reference	Age	Sex	Karyotype
Emadali et al,[32] 2016	3	Jardin et al,[21] 2011 (case 10)	72	Male	49,XY,t(6;8)(p21;q24),+11,+16,+18[19]/46,XY[1]
Emadali et al,[32] 2016	4		41	Male	46,XY,t(6;8)(p21;q24)
Boddu et al,[6] 2018	1	Ohanian et al,[38] 2015 (case 2)	60	Male	46,XY,del(13)(q12q22)[16]/46,idem,t(6;8)(p21;q24.1),del(14)(q24q32)[2]/46,idem,t(6;8)(p21;q24.1),del(14)(q24q32)[cp2]
Boddu et al,[6] 2018	5		71	Male	46,XY,t(6;8)(p21;q24.2)[5]/47,idem,+18[11]/46,XY[4]
Sumarriva Lezama et al,[45] 2018	1		80	Male	75-4n>,XXYY,-1,-3,-4,-5,-5,t(6;8)(p21;q24)x2,-9,-9,-10,-10,-12,-12,-13,-15,-15,-17,-17,-18,-22,-22,+2mar.ish t(6;8)(p21;q24)[17]/46,XY[3]

Only the cases with the full description of the karyotype were listed here.
Abbreviation: wcp, whole chromosome painting.

of MYC-negative and 2/9 (22%) of MYC-indeterminate cases harbored *MYB* rearrangements. This suggested the mutual exclusivity of the functional 8q24 rearrangements resulting in uniform MYC expression and *MYB/MYBL1* rearrangement in BPDCN.

Rearrangements of Other Genes

Sporadic "BPDCN" cases with translocations involving genes other than *MYC* and *MYB* were reported. In an infantile case with a t(2;17;8)(p23;q23;p23) translocation as the sole abnormality shown by karyotyping, a *CLTC-ALK* fusion gene was confirmed by RT-PCR.[53] The clinical presentation of this case was unusual as BPDCN in terms of age and the hemophagocytic lymphohistiocytosis found at diagnosis. The rearrangements of the *MLL* gene, located at 11q23, are commonly found in various types of acute leukemia. Several cases were reported as BPDCN or CD4+/CD56+ hematologic malignancy with *MLL* rearrangements.[54–57] Some cases with rearrangements involving *ETV6* (12p13.2)[12,58] and *EWSR1* (22q12.2)[12,59] were also reported. However, caution is warranted when interpreting the above-mentioned reports because most cases were diagnosed in the era before sufficient pDC-specific markers were available. The diagnoses of these cases could be AML or other hematologic malignancies instead of BPDCN.

SUMMARY

Several recurrent chromosomal deletions involving TSGs, especially the genes regulating the G1/S cell-cycle transition (eg, *CDKN2A*, *CDKN2B*, *CDKN1B*, and *RB1*) were identified in BPDCN. However, the candidate genes in some of the recurrently deleted regions have not been clarified (eg, 6q, 15q). Multiple studies identified chromosome 9, 12p13, and 13q13 as common deleted regions, but there were some regions that showed diverse positive rates among studies, which might reflect the heterogeneity of this disease. The detailed analyses using next-generation sequencing or other newly developed techniques will shed light on those unsolved issues. Recent studies identified recurrent rearrangements of *MYC* and *MYB* family genes in BPDCN. The biological differences among the cases with or without these rearrangements require further elucidation.

DISCLOSURE

The authors have nothing to disclose.

CONFLICT OF INTEREST

The authors declare no potential conflicts of interest regarding this study.

REFERENCES

1. Swerdlow SH, Campo E, Harris NL, et al. WHO classification of tumours of haematopoietic and lymphoid tissues. Revised 4th edition. Lyon (France): IARC; 2017.
2. Facchetti F, Cigognetti M, Fisogni S, et al. Neoplasms derived from plasmacytoid dendritic cells. Mod Pathol 2016;29(2):98–111.
3. Tang Z, Li Y, Wang W, et al. Genomic aberrations involving 12p/ETV6 are highly prevalent in blastic plasmacytoid dendritic cell neoplasms and might represent early clonal events. Leuk Res 2018;73:86–94.

4. Suzuki K, Suzuki Y, Hama A, et al. Recurrent MYB rearrangement in blastic plasmacytoid dendritic cell neoplasm. Leukemia 2017;31(7):1629–33.

5. Sakamoto K, Katayama R, Asaka R, et al. Recurrent 8q24 rearrangement in blastic plasmacytoid dendritic cell neoplasm: association with immunoblastoid cytomorphology, MYC expression, and drug response. Leukemia 2018;32(12):2590–603.

6. Boddu PC, Wang SA, Pemmaraju N, et al. 8q24/MYC rearrangement is a recurrent cytogenetic abnormality in blastic plasmacytoid dendritic cell neoplasms. Leuk Res 2018;66:73–8.

7. Agha ME, Monaghan SA, Swerdlow SH. Venetoclax in a patient with a blastic plasmacytoid dendritic-cell neoplasm. N Engl J Med 2018;379(15):1479–81.

8. Reichard KK, McKenna RW, Kroft SH. ALK-positive diffuse large B-cell lymphoma: report of four cases and review of the literature. Mod Pathol 2007;20(3):310–9.

9. Petrella T, Dalac S, Maynadie M, et al. CD4+ CD56+ cutaneous neoplasms: a distinct hematological entity? Groupe Francais d'Etude des Lymphomes Cutanes (GFELC). Am J Surg Pathol 1999;23(2):137–46.

10. Bayerl MG, Rakozy CK, Mohamed AN, et al. Blastic natural killer cell lymphoma/leukemia: a report of seven cases. Am J Clin Pathol 2002;117(1):41–50.

11. Leroux D. CD4+, CD56+ DC2 acute leukemia is characterized by recurrent clonal chromosomal changes affecting 6 major targets: a study of 21 cases by the Groupe Francais de Cytogenetique Hematologique. Blood 2002;99(11):4154–9.

12. Tang Z, Tang G, Wang SA, et al. Simultaneous deletion of 3′ETV6 and 5′EWSR1 genes in blastic plasmacytoid dendritic cell neoplasm: case report and literature review. Mol Cytogenet 2016;9:23.

13. Mao X, Onadim Z, Price EA, et al. Genomic alterations in blastic natural killer/extranodal natural killer-like T cell lymphoma with cutaneous involvement. J Invest Dermatol 2003;121(3):618–27.

14. Hallermann C, Middel P, Griesinger F, et al. CD4+ CD56+ blastic tumor of the skin: cytogenetic observations and further evidence of an origin from plasmocytoid dendritic cells. Eur J Dermatol 2004;14(5):317–22.

15. Petrella T, Herve G, Bonnotte B, et al. Alpha-interferon secreting blastic plasmacytoid dendritic cells neoplasm: a case report with histological, molecular genetics and long-term tumor cells culture studies. Am J Dermatopathol 2012;34(6):626–31.

16. Oiso N, Tatsumi Y, Arao T, et al. Loss of genomic DNA copy numbers in the p18, p16, p27 and RB loci in blastic plasmacytoid dendritic cell neoplasm. Eur J Dermatol 2012;22(3):393–4.

17. Dijkman R, van Doorn R, Szuhai K, et al. Gene-expression profiling and array-based CGH classify CD4+CD56+ hematodermic neoplasm and cutaneous myelomonocytic leukemia as distinct disease entities. Blood 2007;109(4):1720–7.

18. Jardin F, Callanan M, Penther D, et al. Recurrent genomic aberrations combined with deletions of various tumour suppressor genes may deregulate the G1/S transition in CD4+CD56+ haematodermic neoplasms and contribute to the aggressiveness of the disease. Leukemia 2009;23(4):698–707.

19. Wiesner T, Obenauf AC, Cota C, et al. Alterations of the cell-cycle inhibitors p27(KIP1) and p16(INK4a) are frequent in blastic plasmacytoid dendritic cell neoplasms. J Invest Dermatol 2010;130(4):1152–7.

20. Lucioni M, Novara F, Fiandrino G, et al. Twenty-one cases of blastic plasmacytoid dendritic cell neoplasm: focus on biallelic locus 9p21.3 deletion. Blood 2011; 118(17):4591–4.

21. Jardin F, Ruminy P, Parmentier F, et al. TET2 and TP53 mutations are frequently observed in blastic plasmacytoid dendritic cell neoplasm. Br J Haematol 2011; 153(3):413–6.

22. Kim WY, Sharpless NE. The regulation of INK4/ARF in cancer and aging. Cell 2006;127(2):265–75.

23. Stenzinger A, Endris V, Pfarr N, et al. Targeted ultra-deep sequencing reveals recurrent and mutually exclusive mutations of cancer genes in blastic plasmacytoid dendritic cell neoplasm. Oncotarget 2014;5(15):6404–13.

24. Sapienza MR, Abate F, Melle F, et al. Blastic plasmacytoid dendritic cell neoplasm: genomics mark epigenetic dysregulation as a primary therapeutic target. Haematologica 2019;104(4):729–37.

25. Chu IM, Hengst L, Slingerland JM. The Cdk inhibitor p27 in human cancer: prognostic potential and relevance to anticancer therapy. Nat Rev Cancer 2008;8(4): 253–67.

26. Sherr CJ, Roberts JM. Living with or without cyclins and cyclin-dependent kinases. Genes Dev 2004;18(22):2699–711.

27. Hock H, Shimamura A. ETV6 in hematopoiesis and leukemia predisposition. Semin Hematol 2017;54(2):98–104.

28. Patnaik MM, Lasho T, Howard M, et al. Biallelic inactivation of the retinoblastoma gene results in transformation of chronic myelomonocytic leukemia to a blastic plasmacytoid dendritic cell neoplasm: shared clonal origins of two aggressive neoplasms. Blood Cancer J 2018;8(9):82.

29. Alayed K, Patel KP, Konoplev S, et al. TET2 mutations, myelodysplastic features, and a distinct immunoprofile characterize blastic plasmacytoid dendritic cell neoplasm in the bone marrow. Am J Hematol 2013;88(12):1055–61.

30. Menezes J, Acquadro F, Wiseman M, et al. Exome sequencing reveals novel and recurrent mutations with clinical impact in blastic plasmacytoid dendritic cell neoplasm. Leukemia 2014;28(4):823–9.

31. Fu Y, Fesler M, Mahmud G, et al. Narrowing down the common deleted region of 5q to 6.0 Mb in blastic plasmacytoid dendritic cell neoplasms. Cancer Genet 2013;206(7–8):293–8.

32. Emadali A, Hoghoughi N, Duley S, et al. Haploinsufficiency for NR3C1, the gene encoding the glucocorticoid receptor, in blastic plasmacytoid dendritic cell neoplasms. Blood 2016;127(24):3040–53.

33. Merkenschlager M. Ikaros in immune receptor signaling, lymphocyte differentiation, and function. FEBS Lett 2010;584(24):4910–4.

34. Cytlak U, Resteu A, Bogaert D, et al. Ikaros family zinc finger 1 regulates dendritic cell development and function in humans. Nat Commun 2018;9(1):1239.

35. Mullighan CG, Miller CB, Radtke I, et al. BCR-ABL1 lymphoblastic leukaemia is characterized by the deletion of Ikaros. Nature 2008;453(7191):110–4.

36. Mastio J, Simand C, Cova G, et al. Ikaros cooperates with Notch activation and antagonizes TGFbeta signaling to promote pDC development. PLoS Genet 2018;14(7):e1007485.

37. Tansey WP. Mammalian MYC proteins and cancer. New J Sci 2014;2014:1–27.

38. Ohanian M, Bueso-Ramos C, Ok CY, et al. Acute myeloid leukemia with MYC rearrangement and JAK2 V617F mutation. Cancer Genet 2015;208(11):571–4.

39. Tang G, Hu S, Wang SA, et al. t(3;8)(q26.2;q24) often leads to MECOM/MYC rearrangement and is commonly associated with therapy-related myeloid neoplasms and/or disease progression. J Mol Diagn 2019;21(2):343–51.

40. Momoi A, Toba K, Kawai K, et al. Cutaneous lymphoblastic lymphoma of putative plasmacytoid dendritic cell-precursor origin: two cases. Leuk Res 2002;26(7):693–8.

41. Maeda T, Murata K, Fukushima T, et al. A novel plasmacytoid dendritic cell line, CAL-1, established from a patient with blastic natural killer cell lymphoma. Int J Hematol 2005;81(2):148–54.

42. Takiuchi Y, Maruoka H, Aoki K, et al. Leukemic manifestation of blastic plasmacytoid dendritic cell neoplasm lacking skin lesion: a borderline case between acute monocytic leukemia. J Clin Exp Hematop 2012;52(2):107–11.

43. Nakamura Y, Kayano H, Kakegawa E, et al. Identification of SUPT3H as a novel 8q24/MYC partner in blastic plasmacytoid dendritic cell neoplasm with t(6;8)(p21;q24) translocation. Blood Cancer J 2015;5:e301.

44. Tzankov A, Hebeda K, Kremer M, et al. Plasmacytoid dendritic cell proliferations and neoplasms involving the bone marrow: summary of the workshop cases submitted to the 18th Meeting of the European Association for Haematopathology (EAHP) organized by the European Bone Marrow Working Group, Basel 2016. Ann Hematol 2017;96(5):765–77.

45. Sumarriva Lezama L, Chisholm KM, Carneal E, et al. An analysis of blastic plasmacytoid dendritic cell neoplasm with translocations involving the MYC locus identifies t(6;8)(p21;q24) as a recurrent cytogenetic abnormality. Histopathology 2018;73(5):767–76.

46. Chaperot L. Identification of a leukemic counterpart of the plasmacytoid dendritic cells. Blood 2001;97(10):3210–7.

47. Kurt H, Khoury JD, Medeiros LJ, et al. Blastic plasmacytoid dendritic cell neoplasm with unusual morphology, MYC rearrangement and TET2 and DNMT3A mutations. Br J Haematol 2018;181(3):305.

48. Ceribelli M, Hou ZE, Kelly PN, et al. A druggable TCF4- and BRD4-dependent transcriptional network sustains malignancy in blastic plasmacytoid dendritic cell neoplasm. Cancer Cell 2016;30(5):764–78.

49. Kubota S, Tokunaga K, Umezu T, et al. Lineage-specific RUNX2 super-enhancer activates MYC and promotes the development of blastic plasmacytoid dendritic cell neoplasm. Nat Commun 2019;10(1):1653.

50. George OL, Ness SA. Situational awareness: regulation of the myb transcription factor in differentiation, the cell cycle and oncogenesis. Cancers (Basel) 2014;6(4):2049–71.

51. Brayer KJ, Frerich CA, Kang H, et al. Recurrent fusions in MYB and MYBL1 define a common, transcription factor-driven oncogenic pathway in salivary gland adenoid cystic carcinoma. Cancer Discov 2016;6(2):176–87.

52. Ramkissoon LA, Horowitz PM, Craig JM, et al. Genomic analysis of diffuse pediatric low-grade gliomas identifies recurrent oncogenic truncating rearrangements in the transcription factor MYBL1. Proc Natl Acad Sci U S A 2013;110(20):8188–93.

53. Tokuda K, Eguchi-Ishimae M, Yagi C, et al. CLTC-ALK fusion as a primary event in congenital blastic plasmacytoid dendritic cell neoplasm. Genes Chromosomes Cancer 2014;53(1):78–89.

54. Toya T, Nishimoto N, Koya J, et al. The first case of blastic plasmacytoid dendritic cell neoplasm with MLL-ENL rearrangement. Leuk Res 2012;36(1):117–8.

55. Leung R, Chow EE, Au WY, et al. CD4+/CD56+ hematologic malignancy with rearranged MLL gene. Hum Pathol 2006;37(2):247–9.
56. Bueno C, Almeida J, Lucio P, et al. Incidence and characteristics of CD4(+)/HLA DRhi dendritic cell malignancies. Haematologica 2004;89(1):58–69.
57. Yang N, Huh J, Chung WS, et al. KMT2A (MLL)-MLLT1 rearrangement in blastic plasmacytoid dendritic cell neoplasm. Cancer Genet 2015;208(9):464–7.
58. Gao NA, Wang XX, Sun JR, et al. Blastic plasmacytoid dendritic cell neoplasm with leukemic manifestation and ETV6 gene rearrangement: a case report. Exp Ther Med 2015;9(4):1109–12.
59. Cao Q, Liu F, Niu G, et al. Blastic plasmacytoid dendritic cell neoplasm with EWSR1 gene rearrangement. J Clin Pathol 2014;67(1):90–2.

Chemotherapy Options for Blastic Plasmacytoid Dendritic Cell Neoplasm

Michael Haddadin, MD, Justin Taylor, MD*

KEYWORDS

• BPDCN • Chemotherapy • Induction • Low-intensity

KEY POINTS

• Chemotherapy remains an effective treatment option for BPDCN in fit patients who may be eligible for hematopoietic stem cell transplantation.
• The intensity of induction regimens is positively correlated with outcomes in retrospective series but is difficult to disentangle from possible confounders.
• Some series suggest "ALL-type" or lymphoid-directed regimens are associated with better outcomes compared with "AML-type" or myeloid-directed regimens.
• Low-intensity chemotherapy regimens are of utility in unfit patients who are not eligible to receive novel CD123-targeted therapy.

INTRODUCTION

Blastic plasmacytoid dendritic cell neoplasm (BPDCN) has historically been prone to misdiagnosis and was previously called by several other names, including blastic natural killer (NK) cell tumor and CD4+/CD56+ hematodermic neoplasm,[1,2] which could potentially be the reason there are so many treatment regimens reported in the literature for this disease. Its rarity has also precluded any randomized studies comparing the efficacy of these alternative approaches. The first ever trial solely for BPDCN resulted in the approval of the CD123-targeting immunotoxin tagraxofusp by the Food and Drug Administration (FDA) in 2018.[3] Despite this approval, a consensus approach for the treatment of BPDCN is still lacking. Retrospective data suggest remaining efficacy for induction chemotherapy followed by hematopoietic stem cell transplant in fit patients who are eligible for this approach. In this article, we review the available data for or against certain chemotherapeutic regimens and discuss a

Department of Medicine, Memorial Sloan Kettering Cancer Center, 1275 York Avenue, New York, NY 10065, USA
* Corresponding author.
E-mail address: Taylorj7@mskcc.org
Twitter: @TaylorJ_MD (J.T.)

Hematol Oncol Clin N Am 34 (2020) 539–552
https://doi.org/10.1016/j.hoc.2020.01.011
0889-8588/20/© 2020 Elsevier Inc. All rights reserved.

potential approach that incorporates chemotherapy into algorithms with novel agents and transplant to come up with a logical framework for the treatment of BPDCN.

INTENSIVE CHEMOTHERAPY FOR FIT INDIVIDUALS

Given the lack of prospective trials of induction regimens for BPDCN, the best recommendation for treatments used for induction are based on retrospective analyses of patients treated in routine clinical practice. In our experience, whether the patient was referred to a certain subspecialist influenced the treatment decision.[4] For example, if referred to a lymphoma specialist the patients tended to get lymphoma regimens, for example, CHOP; however, if referred to a leukemia specialist the patients tended to get acute leukemia regimens, such as hyperCVAD or daunorubicin/cytarabine. This would suggest that a comparison of CHOP-like regimens to acute leukemia induction regimens, although limited by the retrospective nature of published studies, might actually be a fair comparison since the only selection of patients occurred at the initial referral level and not due to patient factors that might influence outcomes.

In 2003, Reimer and colleagues[5] collated published data from 97 patients with BPDCN and grouped them into the following categories:

A. Chemotherapy less intensive than CHOP (including local radiotherapy)
B. CHOP and CHOP-like regimens
C. Therapy for acute leukemia
D. Allogeneic/autologous stem cell transplantation

Surprisingly, the overall response rates were no different among the range of intensity of treatments; however, the maintenance of remission was better in the intensive regimen groups and age-adjusted overall survival was superior in the patients with leukemia-based induction regiments followed by allogeneic transplant in first remission (median overall survival = 38.5 months). More recent data from 3 US academic cancer centers also confirmed that the intensity of treatment is associated with improved survival and that BPDCN outcomes likely have improved in the last decade even before novel targeted therapies. For patients receiving intensive regimens (with or without transplant) the 2-year progression-free survival rate was 45%.[4] We have also collated the published data since Reimer's paper, which now include an additional 344 published cases of BPDCN with outcomes data (**Table 1**).

The choice of acute leukemia-based induction regimens seems to vary by institute and even within institutes. The initial categorization of BPDCN in the WHO classification of hematopoietic tumors placed it as a subset of acute myeloid leukemia (AML).[2] Genomic analyses have also recognized that BPDCN harbors many mutations typically seen in myeloid malignancies.[6–10] Therefore, the adoption of AML induction regimens would seem to be logical. Yet multiple retrospective comparisons have shown improved survival with the use of acute lymphoblastic leukemia (ALL)-type induction regimens.[11–13] For example, in 2013, Pagano and colleagues[14] published a series of 41 patients who received either AML-type (63%) or ALL-type (37%) therapies. Seven patients (27%) achieved complete remission (CR) after AML-type therapy and 10 patients (67%) achieved CR after ALL-type therapy with a significant advantage of the lymphoid regimens. The more contemporary experience in the US also showed a trend toward improved survival with lymphoid compared with myeloid regimens.[4]

The reason behind an advantage to lymphoid regimens over myeloid regimens remains unclear. One possibility could be the activity of 1 or multiples of the agents included in ALL-type regimens and the use of L-asparaginase has been proposed

Table 1
Published cases of blastic plasmacytoid dendritic cell neoplasm receiving chemotherapy with outcomes 2003-2019

Authors, Year	n	Chemotherapy	Radiation	No. with Complete Remission	Median Overall Survival (mo)
Kim et al,[33] 2005	6	HyperCVAD (4), ALL-like (2)	N	4	17
Ng et al,[34] 2006	5	CHOP (2), HyperCVAD (1), chlorambucil (1), topical steroids (1)	Y (2)	4/1	26+
Martin et al,[35] 2006	2	CHOP	N	1	6+
Leitenberger et al,[27] 2008	1	CHOP → pralatrexate	N	0	19
Kaune et al,[36] 2009	1	CHOP	N	0	26
Dalle et al,[11] 2010	35	ALL-like (5), AML-like (10), lymphoma (20)	N	18	15.5
Tsagarakis et al,[13] 2010	19	ALL-like (9), AML-like (6), lymphoma (4)	N	15	ND
Tsukune et al,[37] 2010	1	NK/T-like	N	1	14+
Su et al,[38] 2010	2	HyperCVAD	N	0	8
Male et al,[39] 2010	1	Daunorubicin + cytarabine	N	1	18+
Chang et al,[40] 2010	1	NK/T-like	N	0	ND
Li et al,[41] 2011	2	HyperCVAD	N	2	8.5+
Chen et al,[42] 2011	1	Lymphoma-like	N	0	6
Voelkl et al,[43] 2011	1	High-dose cytarabine and mitoxantrone	N	1	26+
Dietrich et al,[44] 2011	6	ALL-like (3), AML-like (2), lymphoma (1)	N	5	16
Lucioni et al,[45] 2011	13	ALL-like (9), lymphoma (4)	N	11	19.8
Steinberg et al,[46] 2011	1	ALL-like	N	1	72+
Inoue et al,[47] 2011	1	Cytarabine and etoposide	N	1	ND
Fukushi et al,[48] 2011	1	NK/T-like	N	1	5
Toya et al,[49] 2012	1	High-dose cytarabine and mitoxantrone	N	1	ND
Dantas et al,[50] 2012	1	CHOP	N	0	2

(continued on next page)

Table 1
(continued)

Authors, Year	n	Chemotherapy	Radiation	No. with Complete Remission	Median Overall Survival (mo)
Rauh et al,[51] 2012	1	CHOP	N	0	9
Munoz et al,[52] 2012	1	Cytarabine and idarubicin	N	0	ND
Wang et al,[53] 2012	1	HyperCVAD	N	1	10
Ham et al,[54] 2012	1	Cytarabine and idarubicin	N	1	24+
Xie et al,[55] 2012	1	CHOP	N	1	24+
Pinto-Almeida et al,[56] 2012	1	Cytarabine and mitoxantrone	N	0	1
Piccin et al,[57] 2012	1	Cytarabine, idarubicin, etoposide	N	1	4
Aoi et al,[58] 2012	1	HyperCVAD	N	1	24+
Takiuchi et al,[59] 2012	1	Cytarabine, etoposide, mitoxantrone	N	1	1
Hashikawa et al,[12] 2012	17	ALL-like (2), AML-like (4), lymphoma (11)	N	11	10
An et al,[60] 2013	6	ALL-like (3), AML-like (1), lymphoma (1)	N	3	5
Unteregger et al,[61] 2013	5	HyperCCVP (3), HyperCVAD (1), CHOPD (1)	N	4	26+
Sanada et al,[62] 2013	1	CHOP	N	1	40+
Pagano et al,[14] 2013	41	AML-like (26), ALL/lymphoma (15)	N	17	10
Ramanathan et al,[63] 2013	1	NK/T-like → AML-like	N	1	10+
Gruson et al,[64] 2013	7	L-Asparaginase, methotrexate, dexamethasone	N	4	18
Alayed et al,[8] 2013	15	HyperCVAD (13), CHOP (2)	N	4	15
Sugimoto et al,[65] 2013	1	NK/T-like	N	1	12+
Borchiellini et al,[66] 2013	4	AML-like (1), lymphoma (3)	N	2	18+
Lencastre et al,[67] 2013	1	CHOP	N	0	7
Goren Sahin et al,[68] 2013	1	Cytarabine, idarubicin, etoposide	N	1	48+
Gera et al,[69] 2014	1	Methotrexate	N	0	8
Dlouhy et al,[70] 2014	1	ALL-like	N	1	24+

Study	Year	N	Treatment			
Chu et al,[71] 2014	2014	2	CHOP (1), no treatment (1)	N	0	2
Starck et al,[72] 2014	2014	1	CHOP	N	0	7
Saeed et al,[73] 2014	2014	1	Cyclophosphamide, vincristine, prednisone	N	1	10
Laribi et al,[23] 2014	2014	2	Azacitidine	N	0	9
Heinicke et al,[74] 2015	2015	9	ALL-like (3), CHOP (5), bexarotene + interferon α (1)	Y (2)	ND	19+
Wang et al,[75] 2015	2015	1	CHOP	N	0	3
Gao et al,[76] 2015	2015	1	CHOP	N	0	7
Yu et al,[77] 2015	2015	1	CHOP	N	0	3
Atalay et al,[78] 2015	2015	3	ALL-like (2), AML-like (1)	N	1	20
Martin-Martin et al,[79] 2015	2015	25	ALL-like (7), AML-like (9), lymphoma (9)	N	23	11+
Kim et al,[80] 2015	2015	6	HyperCVAD (4), other ALL-like (2)	Y (1)	4	17
Deotare et al,[81] 2016	2016	7	HyperCVAD	N	6	35
Khwaja et al,[22] 2016	2016	3	Azacitidine	N	0	19
Arranto et al,[26] 2017	2017	1	Pralatrexate	N	0	5
Ulrickson et al,[25] 2017	2017	3	Gemcitabine and docetaxel (after previous therapies)	N	3	13
Pennisi et al,[82] 2017	2017	1	HyperCVAD	N	1	13+
Barros Ramão et al,[83] 2017	2017	1	HyperCVAD	N	0	5
Bétrian et al,[24] 2017	2017	4	Bendamustine	N	1	25
Kim et al,[84] 2017	2017	3	ALL-like (1), CHOP (1), RT (1)	Y (1)	0	21
Amitay-Laish et al,[85] 2017	2017	2	HyperCVAD and consolidative local RT	Y	2	102+
Fracchiolla et al,[86] 2017	2017	1	Cytarabine and daunorubicin → HyperCVAD	N	0	20
Wang et al,[87] 2018	2018	1	CHOP → ALL-like, maintenance chidamide (HDACi)	N	1	17
Ohe et al,[88] 2018	2018	5	HyperCVAD (4), CHOP (1)	N	ND	33+
Singh et al,[89] 2018	2018	3	ALL-like (2), AML-like (1)	N	2	8+
Yang et al,[90] 2019	2019	1	L-Asparaginase, gemcitabine, oxaliplatin	Y	1	ND (6 mo relapse)
Taylor et al,[4] 2019	2019	44	ALL-like (15), AML-like (7), lymphoma (13), NK/T-like (1), pralatrexate (3), enasidenib, alemtuzumab, decitabine, RT, hydroxyurea (1 each)	Y(1)	30	33+

as a potential explanation,[15] yet many adult ALL regimens do not include L-asparaginase. Another possible explanation could be that ALL regimens incorporate central nervous system (CNS) prophylaxis, which is often not the case in AML regimens. CNS involvement by BPDCN has been described in several studies, with increasing frequency at relapse.[13,14,16] One small study recently demonstrated occult CNS disease at presentation and improved outcome with the addition of intrathecal chemotherapy.[17] These data suggest that, if regimens that do not include CNS coverage are used, CNS prophylaxis should be added. This recommendation could also likely be extended to tagraxofusp since the trial excluded patients with CNS involvement at diagnosis and it is not yet known if CNS relapses will be seen in this setting.

A caveat to all of the above is that with the exception of pediatric BPDCN cases, chemotherapy alone has a low likelihood of producing sustained remissions, and consolidation with hematopoietic stem cell transplantation is required when possible.[18] At present, no studies have looked at the association of measurable residual disease (MRD) levels in patients with BPDCN before transplant and outcomes; however, if extrapolating from data in AML one could assume that MRD positivity would be associated with worse outcomes.[19] This needs to be rigorously evaluated of course, but the presumption would be that more intense regimens are more likely to produce MRD-negative responses and thus better survival when consolidated with stem cell transplant. The specifics of transplant (source, conditioning, graft-versus-host disease prophylaxis, and so forth) are beyond the scope of this article. Although reports from small studies of autologous stem cell transplant are very exciting,[20] larger studies comparing the outcomes of autologous versus allogeneic stem cell transplants are needed before these can be adopted.[21]

Currently, for fit patients when tagraxofusp is not available, the best recommendation is to use intense ALL-type induction regimens followed by allogeneic stem cell transplant. In a modern multicenter analysis of BPDCN outcomes before tagraxofusp was available,[4] the median overall survival of those that were transplanted was 7 years and the survival curve flattened out at about 35%, suggesting long-term survival or cure in a population of patients. Longer-term follow-up is needed for tagraxofusp but, given the high response rates seen in clinical trials and the reduced toxicity compared with intensive induction chemotherapy, tagraxofusp followed by allogeneic transplant in first CR is a reasonable option.

NON-FIT INDIVIDUALS

For patients with BDCN who cannot tolerate aggressive therapy, there is limited data for lower-intensity chemotherapy options. As discussed above, Reimer and colleagues[5] found that those receiving therapies considered less intensive than CHOP had very poor outcomes (median overall survival = 9 months) with only 7% reporting sustained remissions and no patients with long-term survival. The median age in this group was 79 suggesting that they were likely not eligible for hematopoietic stem cell transplant. Tagraxofusp is discussed in more detail by other authors in this series, but suffice it to say this treatment was tolerated in patients and the trial included patients up to the age of 84 years.[3] Notably, 45% of previously untreated patients were consolidated with stem cell transplant in remission, and many of the remainder without transplant also achieved remission and had durable responses. All of these patients had an Eastern Cooperative Oncology Group (ECOG) performance status of 0 or 1, and tagraxofusp may not be tolerated in patients with performance status greater than 2 who were excluded from the trial.

A few small studies have reported outcomes with low-intensity regimens that could be applicable to elderly patients, those with major comorbidities or with an impaired performance status. Two small case series reporting 5 patients in total saw responses to 5-azacitidine that were not long lived[22,23] (median survival = 17 months in 1 series). Bétrian and colleagues[24] observed a response in 1 out of 4 relapsed/refractory patients with BPDCN treated with bendamustine monotherapy where the 1 responder obtained a CR that lasted for 7 months. Another case series of responses observed with low-intensity chemotherapy was reported with the combination of gemcitabine and docetaxel in the relapsed/refractory setting with 2 out of 3 patients achieving CR (median overall survival = 13.3 months).[25] The response rates for these agents might be better if used frontline but further evaluation is needed.

Previous case reports of single-agent pralatrexate, an antifolate chemotherapy, reported partial remissions only[26–28]; however, a recent study that included 8 BPDCN

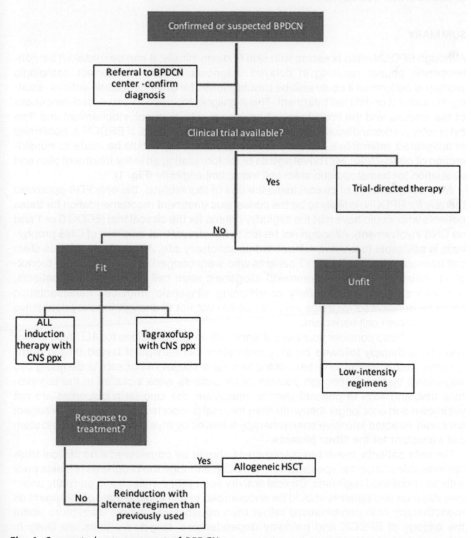

Fig. 1. Suggested management of BPDCN.

patients receiving pralatrexate showed an overall response rate of 75% (6/8) and a complete response rate of 50% (4/8).[4] This included 5 patients treated with relapsed disease. This same study reported 1 patient with an IDH2 mutant BPDCN who achieved blast reduction and stable disease for 8 months on single-agent enasidenib, a mutant IDH2 inhibitor. Based on several reports of responses to treatment with the BCL2 inhibitor, venetoclax,[29–31] single-agent and combination clinical trials are underway.

For patients who are unfit to receive intensive induction chemotherapy and/or hematopoietic stem cell transplant, tagraxofusp should be considered based on fitness. Clinical trials, one of the above less-intensive treatment regimens, or best supportive care can be considered if tagraxofusp is not an option. The development of targeted agents and more tolerable therapies is imperative for this group of patients who currently have the worst outcomes in BPDCN and comprise a substantial proportion of patients with this disease.

SUMMARY

Although BPDCN often presents with skin findings initially, it can be mistaken for non-neoplastic causes resulting in delayed diagnosis. Unless the correct pathologic workup is performed it could also be misdiagnosed for other neoplastic entities resulting in incorrect or delayed treatment. This highlights the need for increased awareness of the disease and the importance of having reliable immunohistochemical and flow cytometry markers, discussed elsewhere in this review series. If BPDCN is confirmed or suspected, referral to a center specializing in this entity should be made for consideration of clinical trials with novel agents or for formulating an initial treatment plan and evaluation for hematopoietic stem cell transplant eligibility (**Fig. 1**).

After consideration of clinical trials, the use of tagraxofusp, the only FDA-approved therapy for BPDCN, is likely to be the consensus treatment recommendation for those patients who would have met the eligibility criteria for the clinical trial (ECOG 0 or 1 and no CNS involvement). Although not tested in the clinical trial, addition of CNS prophylaxis is advisable to prevent relapse in this sanctuary site. Although autologous stem cell transplant was used in 3/13 patients who were bridged to transplant after tagraxofusp initial therapy, we recommend allogeneic stem cell transplant in fit patients. Autologous or reduced intensity conditioning allogeneic stem cell transplantation could be considered for those who are eligible but not fit enough for a myeloablative allogeneic stem cell transplant.

We would also consider younger patients with no comorbidities for ALL-type induction chemotherapy followed by allogeneic stem cell transplant based on the retrospective data showing long-term outcomes for a subset of patients undergoing this aggressive therapy.[4] Although younger adult patients were included in the tagraxofusp trial, and 45% of patients went to transplant, the long-term outcomes are not yet known and until longer follow-up from this trial is reported, we still favor multiagent lymphoid-directed intensive chemotherapy followed by myeloablative allogeneic stem cell transplant for the fittest patients.

For unfit patients, low-intensity regimens should be considered if no clinical trials are available at a center specializing in BPDCN, although the prognosis remains poor with any published regimens. Clinical activity seen with venetoclax is currently under investigation and patients should be encouraged to join clinical trials of this agent as monotherapy or in combinations rather than off-label use. As we learn more about the biology of BPDCN and pathway dependencies, targeted agents are likely to gain a role in treatment of this disease. Anti-CD123-based therapies, such as monoclonal antibodies, bi-specific antibodies, and even CAR-T cells are under development.[32]

Although we hope that rapid transformation in the treatment of BPDCN will bring about a day when cytotoxic chemotherapy is not necessary for any patients, currently there remains a need for it and chemotherapy should be incorporated into algorithms with novel agents and transplant to come up with a multifaceted approach to treatment of BPDCN.

DISCLOSURE

The authors have nothing to disclose.

REFERENCES

1. Adachi M, Maeda K, Takekawa M, et al. High expression of CD56 (N-CAM) in a patient with cutaneous CD4-positive lymphoma. Am J Hematol 1994;47(4): 278–82.

2. Vardiman JW, Thiele J, Arber DA, et al. The 2008 revision of the World Health Organization (WHO) classification of myeloid neoplasms and acute leukemia: rationale and important changes. Blood 2009;114(5):937–51.

3. Pemmaraju N, Lane AA, Sweet KL, et al. Tagraxofusp in blastic plasmacytoid dendritic-cell neoplasm. N Engl J Med 2019;380(17):1628–37.

4. Taylor J, Haddadin M, Upadhyay VA, et al. Multicenter analysis of outcomes in blastic plasmacytoid dendritic cell neoplasm offers a pretargeted therapy benchmark. Blood 2019;134(8):678–87.

5. Reimer P, Rudiger T, Kraemer D, et al. What is CD4+CD56+ malignancy and how should it be treated? Bone Marrow Transplant 2003;32(7):637–46.

6. Menezes J, Acquadro F, Wiseman M, et al. Exome sequencing reveals novel and recurrent mutations with clinical impact in blastic plasmacytoid dendritic cell neoplasm. Leukemia 2014;28(4):823–9.

7. Sapienza MR, Pileri A, Derenzini E, et al. Blastic plasmacytoid dendritic cell neoplasm: state of the art and prospects. Cancers (Basel) 2019;11(5) [pii:E595].

8. Alayed K, Patel KP, Konoplev S, et al. TET2 mutations, myelodysplastic features, and a distinct immunoprofile characterize blastic plasmacytoid dendritic cell neoplasm in the bone marrow. Am J Hematol 2013;88(12):1055–61.

9. Jardin F, Ruminy P, Parmentier F, et al. TET2 and TP53 mutations are frequently observed in blastic plasmacytoid dendritic cell neoplasm. Br J Haematol 2011; 153(3):413–6.

10. Sapienza MR, Fuligni F, Agostinelli C, et al. Molecular profiling of blastic plasmacytoid dendritic cell neoplasm reveals a unique pattern and suggests selective sensitivity to NF-kB pathway inhibition. Leukemia 2014;28(8):1606–16.

11. Dalle S, Beylot-Barry M, Bagot M, et al. Blastic plasmacytoid dendritic cell neoplasm: is transplantation the treatment of choice? Br J Dermatol 2010; 162(1):74–9.

12. Hashikawa K, Niino D, Yasumoto S, et al. Clinicopathological features and prognostic significance of CXCL12 in blastic plasmacytoid dendritic cell neoplasm. J Am Acad Dermatol 2012;66(2):278–91.

13. Tsagarakis NJ, Kentrou NA, Papadimitriou KA, et al. Acute lymphoplasmacytoid dendritic cell (DC2) leukemia: results from the Hellenic Dendritic Cell Leukemia Study Group. Leuk Res 2010;34(4):438–46.

14. Pagano L, Valentini CG, Pulsoni A, et al. Blastic plasmacytoid dendritic cell neoplasm with leukemic presentation: an Italian multicenter study. Haematologica 2013;98(2):239–46.
15. Kerr D 2nd, Zhang L, Sokol L. Blastic plasmacytoid dendritic cell neoplasm. Curr Treat Options Oncol 2019;20(1):9.
16. Feuillard J, Jacob MC, Valensi F, et al. Clinical and biologic features of CD4(+) CD56(+) malignancies. Blood 2002;99(5):1556–63.
17. Martin-Martin L, Almeida J, Pomares H, et al. Blastic plasmacytoid dendritic cell neoplasm frequently shows occult central nervous system involvement at diagnosis and benefits from intrathecal therapy. Oncotarget 2016;7(9):10174–81.
18. Kharfan-Dabaja MA, Reljic T, Murthy HS, et al. Allogeneic hematopoietic cell transplantation is an effective treatment for blastic plasmacytoid dendritic cell neoplasm in first complete remission: systematic review and meta-analysis. Clin Lymphoma Myeloma Leuk 2018;18(11):703–9.e1.
19. Araki D, Wood BL, Othus M, et al. Allogeneic hematopoietic cell transplantation for acute myeloid leukemia: time to move toward a minimal residual disease-based definition of complete remission? J Clin Oncol 2016;34(4):329–36.
20. Aoki T, Suzuki R, Kuwatsuka Y, et al. Long-term survival following autologous and allogeneic stem cell transplantation for blastic plasmacytoid dendritic cell neoplasm. Blood 2015;125(23):3559–62.
21. Kharfan-Dabaja MA, Al Malki MM, Deotare U, et al. Haematopoietic cell transplantation for blastic plasmacytoid dendritic cell neoplasm: a North American multicentre collaborative study. Br J Haematol 2017;179(5):781–9.
22. Khwaja R, Daly A, Wong M, et al. Azacitidine in the treatment of blastic plasmacytoid dendritic cell neoplasm: a report of 3 cases. Leuk Lymphoma 2016;57(11):2720–2.
23. Laribi K, Denizon N, Ghnaya H, et al. Blastic plasmacytoid dendritic cell neoplasm: the first report of two cases treated by 5-azacytidine. Eur J Haematol 2014;93(1):81–5.
24. Bétrian S, Guenounou S, Luquet I, et al. Bendamustine for relapsed blastic plasmacytoid dendritic cell leukaemia. Hematol Oncol 2017;35(2):252–5.
25. Ulrickson ML, Puri A, Lindstrom S, et al. Gemcitabine and docetaxel as a novel treatment regimen for blastic plasmacytoid dendritic cell neoplasm. Am J Hematol 2017;92(5):E75–7.
26. Arranto C, Tzankov A, Halter J. Blastic plasmacytoid dendritic cell neoplasm with transient response to pralatrexate. Ann Hematol 2017;96(4):681–2.
27. Leitenberger JJ, Berthelot CN, Polder KD, et al. CD4+ CD56+ hematodermic/plasmacytoid dendritic cell tumor with response to pralatrexate. J Am Acad Dermatol 2008;58(3):480–4.
28. Sato S, Tanaka E, Tamai Y. Blastic plasmacytoid dendritic cell neoplasm with response to pralatrexate. Ann Hematol 2019;98(3):801–3.
29. DiNardo CD, Rausch CR, Benton C, et al. Clinical experience with the BCL2-inhibitor venetoclax in combination therapy for relapsed and refractory acute myeloid leukemia and related myeloid malignancies. Am J Hematol 2018;93(3):401–7.
30. Montero J, Stephansky J, Cai T, et al. Blastic plasmacytoid dendritic cell neoplasm is dependent on BCL2 and sensitive to venetoclax. Cancer Discov 2017;7(2):156–64.
31. Pemmaraju N, Konopleva M, Lane AA. More on blastic plasmacytoid dendritic-cell neoplasms. N Engl J Med 2019;380(7):695–6.

32. Pemmaraju N. Novel pathways and potential therapeutic strategies for blastic plasmacytoid dendritic cell neoplasm (BPDCN): CD123 and beyond. Curr Hematol Malig Rep 2017;12(6):510–2.

33. Kim Y, Kang MS, Kim CW, et al. CD4+CD56+ lineage negative hematopoietic neoplasm: so called blastic NK cell lymphoma. J Korean Med Sci 2005;20(2): 319–24.

34. Ng AP, Lade S, Rutherford T, et al. Primary cutaneous CD4+/CD56+ hematodermic neoplasm (blastic NK-cell lymphoma): a report of five cases. Haematologica 2006;91(1):143–4.

35. Martín JM, Nicolau MJ, Galan A, et al. CD4+/CD56+ haematodermic neoplasm: a preculsor haematological neoplasm that frequently first presents in the skin. J Eur Acad Dermatol Venereol 2006;20(9):1129–32.

36. Kaune KM, Baumgart M, Bertsch HP, et al. Solitary cutaneous nodule of blastic plasmacytoid dendritic cell neoplasm progressing to overt leukemia cutis after chemotherapy: immunohistology and FISH analysis confirmed the diagnosis. Am J Dermatopathol 2009;31(7):695–701.

37. Tsukune Y, Isobe Y, Yasuda H, et al. Activity and safety of combination chemotherapy with methotrexate, ifosfamide, l-asparaginase and dexamethasone (MILD) for refractory lymphoid malignancies: a pilot study. Eur J Haematol 2010;84(4):310–5.

38. Su O, Onsun N, Demirkesen C, et al. A case of CD4+/CD56+ hematodermic neoplasm (plasmacytoid dendritic cell neoplasm). Dermatol Online J 2010; 16(4):8.

39. Male HJ, Davis MB, McGuirk JP, et al. Blastic plasmacytoid dendritic cell neoplasm should be treated with acute leukemia type induction chemotherapy and allogeneic stem cell transplantation in first remission. Int J Hematol 2010; 92(2):398–400.

40. Chang HJ, Lee MD, Yi HG, et al. A case of blastic plasmacytoid dendritic cell neoplasm initially mimicking cutaneous lupus erythematosus. Cancer Res Treat 2010;42(4):239–43.

41. Li Y, Li Z, Lin HL, et al. Primary cutaneous blastic plasmacytoid dendritic cell neoplasm without extracutaneous manifestation: case report and review of the literature. Pathol Res Pract 2011;207(1):55–9.

42. Chen J, Zhou J, Qin D, et al. Blastic plasmacytoid dendritic cell neoplasm. J Clin Oncol 2011;29(2):e27–9.

43. Voelkl A, Flaig M, Roehnisch T, et al. Blastic plasmacytoid dendritic cell neoplasm with acute myeloid leukemia successfully treated to a remission currently of 26 months duration. Leuk Res 2011;35(6):e61–3.

44. Dietrich S, Andrulis M, Hegenbart U, et al. Blastic plasmacytoid dendritic cell neoplasia (BPDC) in elderly patients: results of a treatment algorithm employing allogeneic stem cell transplantation with moderately reduced conditioning intensity. Biol Blood Marrow Transplant 2011;17(8):1250–4.

45. Lucioni M, Novara F, Fiandrino G, et al. Twenty-one cases of blastic plasmacytoid dendritic cell neoplasm: focus on biallelic locus 9p21.3 deletion. Blood 2011; 118(17):4591–4.

46. Steinberg A, Kansal R, Wong M, et al. Good clinical response in a rare aggressive hematopoietic neoplasm: plasmacytoid dendritic cell leukemia with no cutaneous lesions responding to 4 donor lymphocyte infusions following transplant. Case Rep Transplant 2011;2011:651906.

47. Inoue D, Maruyama K, Aoki K, et al. Blastic plasmacytoid dendritic cell neoplasm expressing the CD13 myeloid antigen. Acta Haematol 2011;126(2):122–8.

48. Fukushi S, Taku F, Aiba S. Blastic plasmacytoid dendritic cell neoplasm on the scalp. Case Rep Dermatol 2011;3(3):240–3.
49. Toya T, Nishimoto N, Koya J, et al. The first case of blastic plasmacytoid dendritic cell neoplasm with MLL-ENL rearrangement. Leuk Res 2012;36(1):117–8.
50. Dantas FE, de Almeida Vieira CA, de Castro CC, et al. Blastic plasmacytoid dendritic cell neoplasm without cutaneous involvement: a rare disease with a rare presentation. Acta Oncol 2012;51(1):139–41.
51. Rauh MJ, Rahman F, Good D, et al. Blastic plasmacytoid dendritic cell neoplasm with leukemic presentation, lacking cutaneous involvement: case series and literature review. Leuk Res 2012;36(1):81–6.
52. Munoz J, Rana J, Inamdar K, et al. Blastic plasmacytoid dendritic cell neoplasm. Am J Hematol 2012;87(7):710.
53. Wang H, Cao J, Hong X. Blastic plasmacytoid dendritic cell neoplasm without cutaneous lesion at presentation: case report and literature review. Acta Haematol 2012;127(2):124–7.
54. Ham JC, Janssen JJ, Boers JE, et al. Allogeneic stem-cell transplantation for blastic plasmacytoid dendritic cell neoplasm. J Clin Oncol 2012;30(8):e102–3.
55. Xie W, Zhao Y, Cao L, et al. Cutaneous blastic plasmacytoid dendritic cell neoplasm occurring after spontaneous remission of acute myeloid leukemia: a case report and review of literature. Med Oncol 2012;29(4):2417–22.
56. Pinto-Almeida T, Fernandes I, Sanches M, et al. A case of blastic plasmacytoid dendritic cell neoplasm. Ann Dermatol 2012;24(2):235–7.
57. Piccin A, Morello E, Svaldi M, et al. Post-transplant lymphoproliferative disease of donor origin, following haematopoietic stem cell transplantation in a patient with blastic plasmacytoid dendritic cell neoplasm. Hematol Oncol 2012;30(4):210–3.
58. Aoi J, Ogata A, Makino T, et al. Case of blastic plasmacytoid dendritic cell neoplasm. J Dermatol 2012;39(12):1066–7.
59. Takiuchi Y, Maruoka H, Aoki K, et al. Leukemic manifestation of blastic plasmacytoid dendritic cell neoplasm lacking skin lesion: a borderline case between acute monocytic leukemia. J Clin Exp Hematop 2012;52(2):107–11.
60. An HJ, Yoon DH, Kim S, et al. Blastic plasmacytoid dendritic cell neoplasm: a single-center experience. Ann Hematol 2013;92(3):351–6.
61. Unteregger M, Valentin A, Zinke-Cerwenka W, et al. Unrelated SCT induces long-term remission in patients with blastic plasmacytoid dendritic cell neoplasm. Bone Marrow Transplant 2013;48(6):799–802.
62. Sanada Y, Nakazato T, Mihara A, et al. Sustained complete remission in an elderly patient with a blastic plasmacytoid dendritic cell neoplasm following autologous peripheral blood stem cell transplantation. Ann Hematol 2013;92(9):1285–6.
63. Ramanathan M, Cerny J, Yu H, et al. A combination treatment approach and cord blood stem cell transplant for blastic plasmacytoid dendritic cell neoplasm. Haematologica 2013;98(3):e36.
64. Gruson B, Vaida I, Merlusca L, et al. L-Asparaginase with methotrexate and dexamethasone is an effective treatment combination in blastic plasmacytoid dendritic cell neoplasm. Br J Haematol 2013;163(4):543–5.
65. Sugimoto KJ, Shimada A, Yamaguchi N, et al. Sustained complete remission of a limited-stage blastic plasmacytoid dendritic cell neoplasm followed by a simultaneous combination of low-dose DeVIC therapy and radiation therapy: a case report and review of the literature. Int J Clin Exp Pathol 2013;6(11):2603–8.
66. Borchiellini D, Ghibaudo N, Mounier N, et al. Blastic plasmacytoid dendritic cell neoplasm: a report of four cases and review of the literature. J Eur Acad Dermatol Venereol 2013;27(9):1176–81.

67. Lencastre A, Cabete J, Joao A, et al. Blastic plasmacytoid dendritic cell neoplasm. An Bras Dermatol 2013;88(6 Suppl 1):158–61.
68. Goren Sahin D, Akay OM, Uskudar Teke H, et al. Blastic plasmacytoid dendritic cell leukemia successfully treated by autologous hematopoietic stem cell transplantation to a remission of 48-month duration. Case Rep Hematol 2013;2013: 471628.
69. Gera S, Dekmezian MS, Duvic M, et al. Blastic plasmacytoid dendritic cell neoplasm: evolving insights in an aggressive hematopoietic malignancy with a predilection of skin involvement. Am J Dermatopathol 2014;36(3):244–51.
70. Dlouhy I, Santacruz R, Pena O. Skin lesions in a patient with blastic plasmacytoid dendritic cell neoplasm. Br J Haematol 2014;164(6):758.
71. Chu G, Verner E, Lee K, et al. Two rare cases of blastic plasmacytoid dendritic cell neoplasm and a literature review. Leuk Lymphoma 2014;55(10):2405–7.
72. Starck M, Zewen S, Eigler A, et al. Meningeal spread of blastic plasmacytoid dendritic cell neoplasm. Eur J Haematol 2014;93(2):175–6.
73. Saeed H, Awasthi M, Al-Qaisi A, et al. Blastic plasmacytoid dendritic cell neoplasm with extensive cutaneous and central nervous system involvement. Rare Tumors 2014;6(4):5474.
74. Heinicke T, Hutten H, Kalinski T, et al. Sustained remission of blastic plasmacytoid dendritic cell neoplasm after unrelated allogeneic stem cell transplantation—a single center experience. Ann Hematol 2015;94(2):283–7.
75. Wang W, Li W, Jia JJ, et al. Blastic plasmacytoid dendritic cell neoplasm: a case report. Oncol Lett 2015;9(3):1388–92.
76. Gao NA, Wang XX, Sun JR, et al. Blastic plasmacytoid dendritic cell neoplasm with leukemic manifestation and ETV6 gene rearrangement: a case report. Exp Ther Med 2015;9(4):1109–12.
77. Yu G, Huang X, Huo Y, et al. Rapid progression of blastic plasmacytoid dendritic cell neoplasm without extracutaneous manifestation. Turk J Haematol 2015; 32(1):98–9.
78. Atalay F, Demirci GT, Bayramgurler D, et al. Blastic plasmacytoid dendritic cell neoplasm: skin and bone marrow infiltration of three cases and the review of the literature. Indian J Hematol Blood Transfus 2015;31(2):302–6.
79. Martín-Martín L, Lopez A, Vidriales B, et al. Classification and clinical behavior of blastic plasmacytoid dendritic cell neoplasms according to their maturation-associated immunophenotypic profile. Oncotarget 2015;6(22):19204–16.
80. Kim JH, Park HY, Lee JH, et al. Blastic plasmacytoid dendritic cell neoplasm: analysis of clinicopathological feature and treatment outcome of seven cases. Ann Dermatol 2015;27(6):727–37.
81. Deotare U, Yee KW, Le LW, et al. Blastic plasmacytoid dendritic cell neoplasm with leukemic presentation: 10-color flow cytometry diagnosis and HyperCVAD therapy. Am J Hematol 2016;91(3):283–6.
82. Pennisi M, Cesana C, Cittone MG, et al. A case of blastic plasmacytoid dendritic cell neoplasm extensively studied by flow cytometry and immunohistochemistry. Case Rep Hematol 2017;2017:4984951.
83. Barros Ramão C, Santos Junior CJD, Leite LAC, et al. Blastic plasmacytoid dendritic cell neoplasm with pulmonary involvement and atypical skin lesion. Am J Case Rep 2017;18:692–5.
84. Kim HS, Kim HJ, Kim SH, et al. Clinical features and treatment outcomes of blastic plasmacytoid dendritic cell neoplasm: a single-center experience in Korea. Korean J Intern Med 2017;32(5):890–9.

85. Amitay-Laish I, Sundram U, Hoppe RT, et al. Localized skin-limited blastic plasmacytoid dendritic cell neoplasm: a subset with possible durable remission without transplantation. JAAD Case Rep 2017;3(4):310–5.

86. Fracchiolla NS, Iurlo A, Ferla V, et al. Concomitant occurrence of blastic plasmacytoid dendritic cell neoplasm and acute myeloid leukaemia after lenalidomide treatment for. Clin Lab 2017;63(9):1513–7.

87. Wang S, Guo W, Wan X, et al. Exploring the effect of chidamide on blastic plasmacytoid dendritic cell neoplasm: a case report and literature review. Ther Clin Risk Manag 2018;14:47–51.

88. Ohe R, Aung NY, Shiono Y, et al. Detection of minimal bone marrow involvement of blastic plasmacytoid dendritic cell neoplastic cells—CD303 immunostaining as a diagnostic tool. J Clin Exp Hematop 2018;58(1):1–9.

89. Singh N, Agrawal N, Agarwal P, et al. Blastic plasmacytoid dendritic cell neoplasm: still an enigma. Indian J Hematol Blood Transfus 2018;34(3):568–72.

90. Yang C, Zhao S, Wang L, et al. Blastic plasmacytoid dendritic cell neoplasm: a case report. Acta Derm Venereol 2019;99(4):456–7.

CD123 as a Therapeutic Target Against Malignant Stem Cells

Mayumi Sugita, MD[a], Monica L. Guzman, PhD[b],*

KEYWORDS

- Acute myeloid leukemia (AML) • Leukemic stem cell (LSC) • BPDCN • CD123
- Targeted therapy

KEY POINTS

- IL-3 receptor α chain (CD123) is aberrantly expressed in leukemia stem cells when compared with its normal counterparts and thus is considered a therapeutic target.
- Identification of unique immunophenotypic features in malignant cells with properties of initiating disease represents a potential avenue for improved outcomes.
- Several immune therapeutic approaches are currently evaluated to eliminate cancer cells expressing CD123.

INTRODUCTION

Cancer stem cells (CSCs) are malignant cells found within tumors, including hematologic malignancies, which possess features associated with normal stem cells such as the ability to self-renew and give rise to progeny such as other tumor cells.[1] In the case of hematologic malignancies, CSCs are best characterized in myeloid malignancies such as myelodysplastic syndrome (MDS), chronic myeloid leukemia (CML), and acute myeloid leukemia (AML). AML is one of the most common acute leukemia in adults with poor prognosis, in the United States it is estimated that around 19,940 new cases will be diagnosed and that 11,180 deaths will occurr in 2020.[2] AML is a hematologic cancer in which abnormal immature myeloid lineage accumulates in the bone marrow. Until very recently, the standard chemotherapy with backbone consisted of the pyrimidine nucleoside analog cytarabine and anthracyclines such as daunorubicin or idarubicin. With this regimen 50% to 80% of patients respond to the initial chemotherapies and enter complete remission. However, most patients relapse and eventually succumb to their disease. Relapses are attributes to the inability of these therapeutic regimens to eliminate LSCs. Despite discoveries of

[a] Division of Hematology and Medical Oncology, Weill Cornell Medical College, 1300 York Avenue, C-660B, New York, NY 10065, USA; [b] Division of Hematology and Medical Oncology, Weill Cornell Medical College, 1300 York Avenue, C-610C, Box 113, New York, NY 10065, USA
* Corresponding author.
E-mail address: mlg2007@med.cornell.edu

Hematol Oncol Clin N Am 34 (2020) 553–564
https://doi.org/10.1016/j.hoc.2020.01.004
0889-8588/20/© 2020 Elsevier Inc. All rights reserved.
hemonc.theclinics.com

very promising therapeutic approaches for AML patients, it is still difficult to maintain AML patients in long-lasting remission.

Increasing efforts in genomic approaches have revealed the heterogeneous mutational landscape in AML that impacts on prognosis and treatment options.[3,4] AML genomes harbor around 10 somatic mutations on average,[5,6] with lower prevalence compared with other adult cancers.[7] The process of leukemogenesis can involve a series of oncogenic events in hematopoietic stem/progenitor cells that can result in a transformed LSC. There is evidence in mouse and human that premalignant HSCs can be found in healthy individuals before the diagnosis of disease or in individuals with AML.[6,8,9] These mutations include DNMT3A, TET2, ASXL1, JAK2, IDH1/2, and TP53.[6,9] Additional mutations in genes such as NPM1, FLT3, RAS, MPL or JAK2 can lead to leukemia.[5] Thus, genomic approaches have also revealed the persistence of malignant clones after therapy (measurable residual disease [MRD]), some with prognostic implications.[10]

Residual disease is often the result of the inability of the therapeutic approach to eliminate all malignant cells, including LSCs. Because of LSCs' stem cell properties, they are capable of leading to disease relapse. Resistance to or evasion of conventional treatments can be attributed to both tumor microenvironment and biological features of LSCs. LSCs of AML were first described as cells capable of initiating human AML after transplantation into severe combined immune deficient (SCID) mice, initially referred as SCID-leukemia initiating cell (SL-ICs).[11] The immunophenotype for these cells was defined as lineage negative (Lin⁻), CD34⁺CD38⁻, shared with HSCs.[12] Patients with high proportions of stem cells have a poor outcome,[13] emphasizing the clinical relevance of these cells.

LSCs reside in the bone marrow (BM) microenvironment and can deprive HSCs from BM niches, limiting their ability to maintain normal hematopoiesis. The BM niche is hypoxic, and provides nutrients and signals that allow LSCs to maintain self-renewal capacity and quiescence features.[14]

Thus, to improve therapeutic outcomes, therapies that can eliminate LSCs without harming normal HSCs are needed. To this end, advances have been made by elucidating features that can distinguish LSCs from HSCs to identify vulnerabilities in LSCs that can be exploited. Some examples of such unique features are unique immunophenotype,[15–18] iron metabolism,[19] amino acid metabolism,[20] epigenetic machinery,[8,21,22] oxidative metabolism,[23] and the epichaperone.[24]

Targeting phenotypic markers, aberrantly expressed antigens on cancer cells, is one highly sought therapeutic approach. Evaluation of phenotypic markers expressed on cells is generally performed by immunohistochemistry (IHC) or multiparameter flow cytometry (MPFC). MPFC technology has enabled interrogation of phenotype of a single cell and has been a powerful and essential tool for diagnosis of hematologic malignancies for monitoring disease. Cancer cells often abnormally express antigens that are not expressed on the normal counterparts, and the information can be used to predict outcomes of disease.

LSCs were first phenotypically defined as Lin⁻/CD34⁺/CD38⁻. With MPFC, key differences in the expression of cell-surface markers between HSCs and LSCs have been evaluated and identified, and some of them represent putative targets against LSCs. Examples of these markers are CD123,[15] CD45RA,[25] C-type lectin-like molecule 1 (CLL1),[26] CD7,[18] CD25,[27] CD44,[28] CD47,[29,30] CD90,[31] CD96,[32] CD99,[33] IL-1RAP,[16] and T cell immunoglobulin and mucin-domain containing-3 (TIM-3).[34] These LSC-specific markers are also being used for disease prognosis and the assessment of MRD.[35] Because of these unique immunophenotypic features, antibody-based therapies or cellular therapies are being developed against some of these antigens. CD123, being the first one identified, is one of most attractive targets, and it is noteworthy that CD123 aberrant expression is found in most patients in blasts, leukemic progenitors, and LSCs.[36]

CD123 IN NORMAL HEMATOPOIETIC CELLS AND NORMAL TISSUES

Interleukin-3 receptor α chain (IL-3RA or CD123) is expressed in basophils, dendritic cells, monocytes, myeloid progenitors of normal hematopoietic cells, and endothelial cells.[37–43] IL-3R is a transmembrane and heterodimeric receptor consisting of α subunit specific to IL-3 and β subunit shared by receptors for interleukin-5 (IL-5) and granulocyte-macrophage colony-stimulating factor (GM-CSF).[44–46] Even though the α subunit itself has a low affinity to IL-3, IL-3R gains high affinity to IL-3 by forming a heterodimeric receptor with common β subunit that works as a main transmitter of signaling. Binding of IL-3 to IL-3R initiates antiapoptotic and cell-proliferative signals through activation of signal transducer and activator of transcription proteins.

CD123 EXPRESSION IN MALIGNANCIES

In malignancies, CD123 is abnormally expressed in AML,[36,47,48] a subtype of hairy cell leukemia,[47–49] MDS,[50] CML,[51] and blastic plasmacytoid dendritic cell neoplasm (BPDCN),[52] and a subset of B-acute lymphoblastic leukemias (B-ALL)[47,53,54] and T-ALL,[55,56] or Hodgkin lymphoma.[57,58] As mentioned earlier, in AML CD123 can be found in blasts, CD34+ progenitors, and CD34+CD38− LSCs, whereas normal HSCs have little (less than 1%) to no CD123 expression.[15,40,47,48,59]

Novel tumor-specific antigens progressively identified in the last 2 decades urged the development of antibody therapies such as monoclonal antibody, bispecific T cell engagers (BiTEs), or antibody-drug conjugates (ADC), and cellular therapies such as chimeric antigen receptor (CAR) T cells. Targeting tumor cell-surface antigens allows antibodies or cytotoxic T cells to detect targeted molecules directly expressed on the cell surface. All of these approaches are being or have been pursued for CD123.

Tagraxofusp

Tagraxofusp (SL-401) is a CD123-targeted recombinant fusion protein consisting of IL-3 and truncated diphtheria toxin (DT).[60] The IL-3 domain of SL-401 dominantly binds to IL-3R with high specificity on CD123+ cells followed by internalization of SL-401 and catalytic domain of truncated DT inhibits protein synthesis to induce cell death. In preclinical studies, SL-401 demonstrated high activity against AML/MDS progenitors and LSCs that are expressing CD123; however, it also showed activity against normal cord blood and normal marrow progenitors in vitro and in patient-derived xenograft models.[61] This result suggests that SL-401 has the potential to eliminate LSCs, and it is currently under evaluation in a phase 1/2 study for AML and MDS patients (NCT00397579).

In addition to a potential toxicity of normal hematopoiesis in preclinical setting, the acquisition of resistance to SL-401 in AML/BPDCN caused by impairment of diphthamide synthesis that is mediated by an enzyme encoded by DPH1 gene was reported.[62] DPH1 gene expression was downregulated through DNA CpG methylation in SL-401 resistant cells and DPH1 expression, and SL-401 sensitivity was restored by azacitidine, a DNA methyltransferase inhibitor, in patient-derived xenograft (PDX) models.[62] A phase 1 clinical trial of a combination of SL-401 and azacitidine or azacitidine/venetoclax for refractory AML or high-risk MDS patients is ongoing (NCT03113643).

Bispecific Antibodies

A bispecific antibody is an antibody harboring 2 or more antigen-recognition sites by combining 2 or more antibodies formed into a single construct that allows to bind to multiple targets simultaneously. Several formats for bispecific antibodies have been developed in the past decade, such as BiTEs, dual-affinity retargeting proteins (DARTs), and tandem diabodies.[63–66]

Flotetuzumab (MGD006) was developed to target CD123 and CD3 (CD123×CD3 DART). In preclinical PDX models injected with primary AML cells and endogenous T cells in tumor samples with low E:T ratio, flotetuzumab significantly reduced leukemia burden in PDX through T cell mediation.[67] A phase 1 clinical trial for patients with relapsed/refractory AML reported that flotetuzumab benefited primary refractory AML patients with a complete response (CR) rate of 29.4% (5/17) with manageable mild/moderate cytokine release syndrome events (NCT02152956).[68] The phase 2 clinical trial for recurrent and refractory CD123-positive blood cancer is under way (NCT03739606).

Antibody-Drug Conjugates

Gemtuzumab ozogamicin is an example of a recombinant monoclonal antibody (mAb)-drug conjugate (ADC) consisting of an anti-CD33 conjugated to a calicheamicin derivative. It is approved by the US Food and Drug Administration (FDA) for adult patients with newly diagnosed CD33$^+$ AML and pediatric patients 2 years or older with relapse/refractory CD33$^+$ AML. Early progenitors of AML and LSCs express very low levels of CD33; thus a similar approach has been used to develop ADC directed to LSC markers such as CD123. One example is IMGN632, an ADC conjugated with an alkylating monoamine containing indolinobenzodiazepine pseudodimer (IGN) molecules. IMGN632 harbors a humanized antibody, G4723A, that binds to the D2-D3 region of extracellular domain of CD123, which allows targeting of both full-length CD123 and an alternative splicing variant that lacks an N-terminal domain[69] but the remaining D2-D3 domain without affecting normal cells with lower levels of CD123 expression.[70] A preclinical study demonstrated the activity of IMGN632 against AML with a lower dose than affects normal hematopoietic cells in vivo and in vitro.[70] Based on the preclinical results, a phase 1 dose-escalation study of IMGN632 for patients with relapsed/refractory AML and other CD123$^+$ hematologic malignancies is ongoing (NCT03386513).

Antibody-Dependent Cell-Mediated Cytotoxicity

7G3 is a mouse mAb that binds to the N-terminal domain of IL-3RA.[71] 7G3 diminished IL-3R biological activity of primary AML cells in vitro dose dependently under exogenous IL-3 stimulation and inhibited proliferation of AML cell lines.[40] In vivo, 7G3 eliminated LSCs in BM and activated innate immunity in NOD/SCID mice resulting in reduced engraftment of AML, but not that of BM in NOD/SCID mice.[40] Additionally CSL360, a 7G3-derived immunoglobulin G$_1$ (IgG$_1$) recombinant chimeric antibody with identical antagonizing activity in IL-3 signaling, did not affect any hematologic parameters in a toxicology study in nonhuman primates.[40] However, in the phase 1 study of CSL360 for relapsed/refractory AML patients, CSL360 did not induce anti-AML activity in most patients[72] (NCT00401739). The same group developed a fully humanized anti-CD123 mAb, CSL362, by engineering the Fc domain of CSL360 to enhance affinity with FcγRIIIa (CD16) on natural killer cells, resulting in induction of ADCC.[73] The activity of CSL362 on AML in vitro and in vivo has been shown in a preclinical study, supporting the clinical development of CSL362 for the treatment of AML patients.[73–77]

CSL362 is currently under evaluation in a phase 2/3 study in combination with decitabine (NCT02472145).

Chimeric Antigen Receptor T Cells

One of new approaches against cancers is the use of cellular therapy such as chimeric antigen receptor (CAR) T cell therapy. The successful CAR T cell therapy targeting CD19 (CD19 CAR T) has shown that these cells are highly effective and induce durable remission in relapsed/refractory B cell acute lymphoblastic leukemia (ALL) patients in the last few years. The approval of first cellular immunotherapy by the FDA in 2017 for Kymriah (tisagenlecleucel) in pediatric/young adult ALL and Yescarta (axicabtagene ciloleucel) in adult non-Hodgkin lymphoma have laid new paths for patients with recurrent/refractory cancer and health care providers. CAR-based approaches against AML and other cancers have been explored to follow the success of CD19 CAR T.

Like targeted-antibody–based therapies, LSC-specific antigens are candidates as targets for CAR T therapy to achieve long remission and potential cure. CD123 is a desirable candidate for CAR T–based treatment against AML. Several CAR T studies targeting CD123 (CD123 CAR T) have shown encouraging results in vitro and in preclinical in vivo settings.[78–81] Preclinical models have shown potent antileukemia activity in primary patient-derived AML xenograft model (PDX-AML).[59,81] Regardless of levels of CD123 at baseline, CART123 cleared engrafted AML rapidly from PDX animals. However, a xenograft model engrafted with normal human CD34+ cells showed impairment of normal human hematopoiesis.[59] Other groups have also demonstrated the antitumor effect of CD123-specific CAR T against AML in vitro and in vivo.[79] These "CD123-specific CAR T cells" were later developed as a drug called MB-102, for which currently the phase 1 clinical trial of patients with relapsed/refractory AML and persistent/refractory BPDCN is ongoing (NCT02159495).

Allogeneic approaches for CAR T therapies referred to as "off-the-shelf" or "universal" CAR T cells (UCAR T) have been developed by using healthy donor T cells. CAR-transduced T cells are engineered to have knocked out T cell receptors to prevent graft-versus-host-disease and off-target cytotoxicity by UCAR T toward normal recipient tissues. UCAR T cell therapy can be a salvage method for patients who are not able to harvest their normal T cells to generate CAR T. In AML, UCAR T targeting CD123 (UCART123) was reported to have anti-AML activity in vitro with minimum effect on normal CD34+ cells.[82] This UCART123 also eliminated AML cells with significant benefits in overall survival in a PDX-AML model and was demonstrated to target preferentially AML cells in a competitive normal BM/AML model. A phase 1 clinical trial of auto-CAR T for refractory AML (NCT03766126) and a phase 1 trial of UCART123 for patients with relapsed/refractory AML (NCT03190278) are ongoing.

The relevance of these strategies is that the impact of other malignancies that overexpress CD123 in different malignant compartments may benefit from this approach, including BPDCN. CD123 CAR T cells have been also used to overcome an immunosuppressive tumor microenvironment in Hodgkin lymphoma.[83]

CD123 TARGETING IN OTHER MALIGNANCIES

As CD123 has been found to be aberrantly expressed in other hematologic malignancies, therapeutic approaches targeting CD123 have been evaluated, including MDS, ALL, lymphoma, and BPDCN.

MDS is a clonal hematopoietic disorder with BM failure that arises from HSCs with one or more genomic mutations, whereby MDS stem cells (MDS-SCs) have been defined and characterized. Recently MDS-SCs were phenotypically defined as

$Lin^-CD34^+CD38^-CD90^+CD45RA^-$,[84] and propagated MDS in NSG mice. Importantly, CD123 was identified in $Lin^-CD34^+CD38^-$ in stem cell compartments. Such a population of cells was demonstrated to have distinct biological features with hyperactivated protein synthesis and increased oxidative phosphorylation when compared with $Lin^-CD34^+CD38^-CD123^-$ cells.[50] Given the role of MDS-SCs, it has been hypothesized that targeting $CD123^+$ MDS-SCs is a rational approach for treatment of high-risk MDS. Phase 1/2 clinical trials for CD123-targeted therapies such as SL-401 (NCT00397579), flotetuzumab (MGD006, NCT02152956), and MB-102 (NCT04109482) for patients with high-risk MDS along with relapsed/refractory AML have been performed or are ongoing. Evaluation of efficacy of these targeted therapies in MDS patients may require accumulation of clinical data.

Even with the emergence and approvals of CD19-targeted immunotherapies for B-ALL, there is interest to further improve therapeutic approaches for these relapse/refractory patients given that CD19-negative relapses can occur.[85,86] CD123 is aberrantly expressed in a subset of B-ALL patients in blasts and LSCs (or leukemia-initiating cells) defined as $CD34^+CD38^-$ capable of propagating B-ALL in NSG mice. It was also found that CD123 was retained in CD19-negative cells in relapsed patient samples. Thus, CAR T targeting CD123 (CART123) was evaluated and found it that could eliminate CD19-negative leukemia. Importantly a dual CD19- and CD123-targeted CAR T successfully prevented relapse with loss of CD19 in a PDX model with relapsed B-ALL blasts.[87] CD123-targeted therapy combined with CD19-directed therapies is a promising approach to eliminate $CD123^+$ B-ALL stem cells.

Classic Hodgkin lymphoma (cHL) is a neoplasm derived from germinal center B cells. Combination of chemotherapy with radiotherapy has achieved prolonged survival in about 80% of cHL patients; however, 20% to 30% with advanced-stage disease are refractory to first-line therapy or relapse with poor prognosis. cHL is composed of 1% to 2% neoplastic Hodgkin Reed-Sternberg (H-RS) cells. In cHL, the tumor environment (TME) cells consist of infiltrating immune cells such as macrophages and myeloid-derived suppressor cells (MDSCs), inflammatory B cells and T cells, mast cells, eosinophils, plasma cells, stromal cells, and fibroblasts.[83] H-RS cells and TME have been shown to play a critical role in tumor progression. CD123 is expressed on 60% to greater than 90% of H-RS cells,[57,83,88] tumor-associated macrophages (TAMs),[57,83] and MDSCs[89] in the tumor site. The CD123-targeting CAR T strategy demonstrated activity against an HL cell line using a xenograft model. Importantly, using a macrophage-killing assay, CD123-targeting CAR T cells were capable of eliminating induced-M2 macrophages and their proliferation was not affected, in contrast to the control CD19 CAR T cells, which were significantly suppressed by induced-M2 macrophages.[83] Thus, in this case targeting CD123 is an immunomodulatory intervention in TME cells and represents a promising approach that may be relevant for other malignancies.

Finally, one more malignancy where targeting CD123 is highly relevant is BPDCN. In preclinical studies, SL-401 demonstrated antitumor activity against BPDCN cell lines both in vitro and in a xenograft mouse model engrafted with BPDCN cell lines.[90] In a pilot study of SL-401 for BPDCN (NCT00397579), 78% of BPDCN patients (7 of 9 evaluable patients) responded to SL-401 including 5 complete responses and 2 partial responses after the first course.[91] The subsequent phase 1/2 study of SL-401 (tagraxofusp) for BPDCN and AML patients (NCT02113982) demonstrated robust activity of SL-401 with 90% overall response rate (26 of 29 evaluable patients) and 72% CR rate (21 of 29) in first-line BPDCN, and 67% overall response rate (10 of 15) in previously treated patients.[92] Based on the results of this study, SL-401 was approved as a first-line and a salvage therapeutic drug for BPDCN by the FDA. Based on encouraging data of SL-401 and antibody-based therapies targeting CD123, and CAR T–based approaches are also currently being evaluated including allogeneic CAR T cells.[93] (NCT03203369) Even though a CSC has not been yet evaluated in BPDCN, the important role of CD123 in other CSCs warrants such studies.

SUMMARY

CD123, IL-3 receptor α chain (IL-3RA), is aberrantly expressed in several hematologic malignancies including MDS, CML, AML, BPDCN, ALL, and Hodgkin lymphoma, in tumor cells or in the tumor microenvironment. Importantly, CD123 is found in CSCs, which are not effectively eliminated by chemotherapy, have the capacity to self-renew, and are capable recapitulating disease. Thus, approaches to target are highly sought and have been tested in preclinical and clinical settings. While the clinical use of approaches targeting CD123 is in progress, it remains of interest to determine whether eradication of the cells capable of imitating and maintaining tumors can be achieved.

DISCLOSURE

M.L. Guzman reports receiving research funding (R01 CA234478) from NIH. M.L. Guzman receives research funding from Cellectis and and honoraria from SeqRx. M. Sugita has nothing to disclose.

REFERENCES

1. Batlle E, Clevers H. Cancer stem cells revisited. Nat Med 2017;23(10):1124–34.

2. Available at: Cancer.net. Accessed January, 2020.

3. Ley TJ, Miller C, Ding L, et al. Genomic and Epigenomic landscapes of adult De Novo Acute Myeloid Leukemia. N Engl J Med 2013;368(22):2059–74.

4. Papaemmanuil E, Gerstung M, Bullinger L, et al. Genomic classification and prognosis in acute myeloid leukemia. N Engl J Med 2016;374(23):2209–21.

5. Welch JS, Ley TJ, Link DC, et al. The origin and evolution of mutations in acute myeloid leukemia. Cell 2012;150(2):264–78.

6. Desai P, Mencia-Trinchant N, Savenkov O, et al. Somatic mutations precede acute myeloid leukemia years before diagnosis. Nat Med 2018;24(7):1015–23.

7. Alexandrov LB, Nike-Zainal S, Wedge DC, et al. Signatures of mutational processes in human cancer. Nature 2013;500(7463):415–21.

8. Shlush LI, Zandi S, Mitchell A, et al. Identification of pre-leukaemic haematopoietic stem cells in acute leukaemia. Nature 2014;506(7488):328–33.

9. Abelson S, Collord G, Ng SWK, et al. Prediction of acute myeloid leukaemia risk in healthy individuals. Nature 2018;559(7714):400–4.

10. Jongen-Lavrencic M, Hanekamp TGD, Kavelaars FG, et al. Molecular minimal residual disease in acute myeloid leukemia. N Engl J Med 2018;378(13):1189–99.

11. Lapidot T, Sirard C, Vormoor J, et al. A cell initiating human acute myeloid leukaemia after transplantation into SCID mice. Nature 1994;367(6464):645–8.

12. Bonnet D, Dick JE. Human acute myeloid leukemia is organized as a hierarchy that originates from a primitive hematopoietic cell. Nat Med 1997;3(7):730–7.

13. van Rhenen A, Feller N, Kelder A, et al. High stem cell frequency in acute myeloid leukemia at diagnosis predicts high minimal residual disease and poor survival. Clin Cancer Res 2005;11(18):6520–7.

14. Ishikawa F, Yoshida S, Saito Y, et al. Chemotherapy-resistant human AML stem cells home to and engraft within the bone-marrow endosteal region. Nat Biotechnol 2007;25(11):1315–21.

15. Jordan CT, Upchurch D, Szilvassy SJ, et al. The interleukin-3 receptor alpha chain is a unique marker for human acute myelogenous leukemia stem cells. Leukemia 2000;14(10):1777–84.

16. Barreyro L, Will B, Bartholdy B, et al. Overexpression of IL-1 receptor accessory protein in stem and progenitor cells and outcome correlation in AML and MDS. Blood 2012;120(6):1290–8.

17. Majeti R, Park CY, Weissman IL. Identification of a hierarchy of multipotent hematopoietic progenitors in human cord blood. Cell Stem Cell 2007;1(6):635–45.

18. van Rhenen A, Moshaver B, Kelder A, et al. Aberrant marker expression patterns on the CD34+CD38- stem cell compartment in acute myeloid leukemia allows to distinguish the malignant from the normal stem cell compartment both at diagnosis and in remission. Leukemia 2007;21(8):1700–7.

19. Trujillo-Alonso V, Pratt EC, Zong H, et al. FDA-approved ferumoxytol displays anti-leukaemia efficacy against cells with low ferroportin levels. Nat Nanotechnol 2019;14(6):616–22.

20. Jones CL, Stevens BM, D'Alessandro A, et al. Inhibition of amino acid metabolism selectively targets human leukemia stem cells. Cancer Cell 2018;34(5):724–740 e4.

21. Corces-Zimmerman MR, Hong WJ, Weissman IL, et al. Preleukemic mutations in human acute myeloid leukemia affect epigenetic regulators and persist in remission. Proc Natl Acad Sci U S A 2014;111(7):2548–53.

22. Jan M, Snyder TM, Corces-Zimmerman MR, et al. Clonal evolution of preleukemic hematopoietic stem cells precedes human acute myeloid leukemia. Sci Transl Med 2012;4(149):149ra118.

23. Lagadinou ED, Sach A, Callahan K, et al. BCL-2 inhibition targets oxidative phosphorylation and selectively eradicates quiescent human leukemia stem cells. Cell Stem Cell 2013;12(3):329–41.

24. Zong H, Gozman A, Caldas-Lopes E, et al. A hyperactive signalosome in acute myeloid leukemia drives addiction to a tumor-specific Hsp90 species. Cell Rep 2015;13(10):2159–73.

25. Kersten B, Valkering M, Wouters R, et al. CD45RA, a specific marker for leukaemia stem cell sub-populations in acute myeloid leukaemia. Br J Haematol 2016;173(2):219–35.

26. van Rhenen A, van Dongen GA, Kelder A, et al. The novel AML stem cell associated antigen CLL-1 aids in discrimination between normal and leukemic stem cells. Blood 2007;110(7):2659–66.

27. Saito Y, Kitamura H, Tomizawa-Murasawa M, et al. Identification of therapeutic targets for quiescent, chemotherapy-resistant human leukemia stem cells. Sci Transl Med 2010;2(17):17ra9.

28. Jin L, Hope KJ, Zhai Q, et al. Targeting of CD44 eradicates human acute myeloid leukemic stem cells. Nat Med 2006;12(10):1167–74.

29. Jaiswal S, Jamieson CH, Pang WW, et al. CD47 is upregulated on circulating hematopoietic stem cells and leukemia cells to avoid phagocytosis. Cell 2009;138(2):271–85.

30. Majeti R, Chao MP, Alizadeh AA, et al. CD47 is an adverse prognostic factor and therapeutic antibody target on human acute myeloid leukemia stem cells. Cell 2009;138(2):286–99.

31. Blair A, Hogge DE, Ailles LE, et al. Lack of expression of Thy-1 (CD90) on acute myeloid leukemia cells with long-term proliferative ability in vitro and in vivo. Blood 1997;89(9):3104–12.

32. Hosen N, Park CY, Tatsumi N, et al. CD96 is a leukemic stem cell-specific marker in human acute myeloid leukemia. Proc Natl Acad Sci U S A 2007;104(26): 11008–13.

33. Chung SS, Eng WS, Hu W, et al. CD99 is a therapeutic target on disease stem cells in myeloid malignancies. Sci Transl Med 2017;9(374).

34. Kikushige Y, Shima T, Takayanagi S, et al. TIM-3 is a promising target to selectively kill acute myeloid leukemia stem cells. Cell Stem Cell 2010;7(6):708–17.

35. Zeijlemaker W, Kelder A, Oussoren-Brockhoff YJ, et al. A simple one-tube assay for immunophenotypical quantification of leukemic stem cells in acute myeloid leukemia. Leukemia 2016;30(2):439–46.

36. Cruz NM, Sugita M, Ewing-Crystal N, et al. Selection and characterization of antibody clones are critical for accurate flow cytometry-based monitoring of CD123 in acute myeloid leukemia. Leuk Lymphoma 2018;59(4):978–82.

37. Olweus J, BitMansour A, Warnke R, et al. Dendritic cell ontogeny: a human dendritic cell lineage of myeloid origin. Proc Natl Acad Sci U S A 1997;94(23): 12551–6.

38. Han X, Jorgensen JL, Brahmandam A, et al. Immunophenotypic study of basophils by multiparameter flow cytometry. Arch Pathol Lab Med 2008;132(5):813–9.

39. Masten BJ, Olson GK, Tarleton CA, et al. Characterization of myeloid and plasmacytoid dendritic cells in human lung. J Immunol 2006;177(11):7784–93.

40. Jin L, Lee EM, Ramshaw HS, et al. Monoclonal antibody-mediated targeting of CD123, IL-3 receptor alpha chain, eliminates human acute myeloid leukemic stem cells. Cell Stem Cell 2009;5(1):31–42.

41. Florian S, Sonneck K, Hasuwirth AW, et al. Detection of molecular targets on the surface of CD34+/CD38– stem cells in various myeloid malignancies. Leuk Lymphoma 2006;47(2):207–22.

42. Korpelainen EI, Gamble JR, Vadas MA, et al. IL-3 receptor expression, regulation and function in cells of the vasculature. Immunol Cell Biol 1996;74(1):1–7.

43. Taussig DC, Pearce DJ, Simposon C, et al. Hematopoietic stem cells express multiple myeloid markers: implications for the origin and targeted therapy of acute myeloid leukemia. Blood 2005;106(13):4086–92.

44. Kitamura T, Sato N, Arai K, et al. Expression cloning of the human IL-3 receptor cDNA reveals a shared beta subunit for the human IL-3 and GM-CSF receptors. Cell 1991;66(6):1165–74.

45. Bagley CJ, Woodcock JM, Stomski FC, et al. The structural and functional basis of cytokine receptor activation: lessons from the common beta subunit of the granulocyte-macrophage colony-stimulating factor, interleukin-3 (IL-3), and IL-5 receptors. Blood 1997;89(5):1471–82.

46. Guthridge MA, Stomski FC, Thomas D, et al. Mechanism of activation of the GM-CSF, IL-3, and IL-5 family of receptors. Stem Cells 1998;16(5):301–13.

47. Munoz L, Nomdedeu JF, Lopez O, et al. Interleukin-3 receptor alpha chain (CD123) is widely expressed in hematologic malignancies. Haematologica 2001;86(12):1261–9.

48. Testa U, Riccioni R, Militi S, et al. Elevated expression of IL-3Ralpha in acute myelogenous leukemia is associated with enhanced blast proliferation, increased cellularity, and poor prognosis. Blood 2002;100(8):2980–8.

49. Del Giudice I, Matutes E, Morilla R, et al. The diagnostic value of CD123 in B-cell disorders with hairy or villous lymphocytes. Haematologica 2004;89(3):303–8.

50. Stevens BM, Khan N, D'Alessandro A, et al. Characterization and targeting of malignant stem cells in patients with advanced myelodysplastic syndromes. Nat Commun 2018;9(1):3694.

51. Nievergall E, Ramshaw HS, Young AS, et al. Monoclonal antibody targeting of IL-3 receptor alpha with CSL362 effectively depletes CML progenitor and stem cells. Blood 2014;123(8):1218–28.

52. Hwang K, Park CJ, Jang S, et al. Immunohistochemical analysis of CD123, CD56 and CD4 for the diagnosis of minimal bone marrow involvement by blastic plasmacytoid dendritic cell neoplasm. Histopathology 2013;62(5):764–70.

53. Hassanein NM, Alcancia F, Perkinson KR, et al. Distinct expression patterns of CD123 and CD34 on normal bone marrow B-cell precursors ("hematogones") and B lymphoblastic leukemia blasts. Am J Clin Pathol 2009;132(4):573–80.

54. Djokic M, Björklund E, Blennow E, et al. Overexpression of CD123 correlates with the hyperdiploid genotype in acute lymphoblastic leukemia. Haematologica 2009;94(7):1016–9.

55. Lhermitte L, de Labarthe A, Dupret C, et al. Most immature T-ALLs express Ra-IL3 (CD123): possible target for DT-IL3 therapy. Leukemia 2006;20(10):1908–10.

56. Angelova E, Audette C, Kovtun Y, et al. CD123 expression patterns and selective targeting with a CD123-targeted antibody-drug conjugate (IMGN632) in acute lymphoblastic leukemia. Haematologica 2019;104(4):749–55.

57. Fromm JR. Flow cytometric analysis of CD123 is useful for immunophenotyping classical Hodgkin lymphoma. Cytometry B Clin Cytom 2011;80(2):91–9.

58. Liu K, Zhu M, Huang Y, et al. CD123 and its potential clinical application in leukemias. Life Sci 2015;122:59–64.

59. Gill S, Tasian SK, Ruella M, et al. Preclinical targeting of human acute myeloid leukemia and myeloablation using chimeric antigen receptor-modified T cells. Blood 2014;123(15):2343–54.

60. Frankel A, Liu JS, Rizzieri D, et al. Phase I clinical study of diphtheria toxin-interleukin 3 fusion protein in patients with acute myeloid leukemia and myelodysplasia. Leuk Lymphoma 2008;49(3):543–53.

61. Mani R, Goswami S, Gopalakrishnan B, et al. The interleukin-3 receptor CD123 targeted SL-401 mediates potent cytotoxic activity against CD34(+)CD123(+) cells from acute myeloid leukemia/myelodysplastic syndrome patients and healthy donors. Haematologica 2018;103(8):1288–97.

62. Togami K, Pastika T, Stephansky J, et al. DNA methyltransferase inhibition overcomes diphthamide pathway deficiencies underlying CD123-targeted treatment resistance. J Clin Invest 2019;129(11):5005–19.

63. Topp MS, Kufer P, Gokbüget N, et al. Targeted therapy with the T-cell-engaging antibody blinatumomab of chemotherapy-refractory minimal residual disease in B-lineage acute lymphoblastic leukemia patients results in high response rate and prolonged leukemia-free survival. J Clin Oncol 2011;29(18):2493–8.

64. Chichili GR, Huang L, Li H, et al. A CD3xCD123 bispecific DART for redirecting host T cells to myelogenous leukemia: preclinical activity and safety in nonhuman primates. Sci Transl Med 2015;7(289):289ra82.

65. Friedrich M, Henn A, Raum T, et al. Preclinical characterization of AMG 330, a CD3/CD33-bispecific T-cell-engaging antibody with potential for treatment of acute myelogenous leukemia. Mol Cancer Ther 2014;13(6):1549–57.

66. Reusch U, Harrington KH, Gudgeon CJ, et al. Characterization of CD33/CD3 tetravalent bispecific tandem diabodies (TandAbs) for the treatment of acute myeloid leukemia. Clin Cancer Res 2016;22(23):5829–38.

67. Al-Hussaini M, Retting MP, Ritchey JK, et al. Targeting CD123 in acute myeloid leukemia using a T-cell-directed dual-affinity retargeting platform. Blood 2016; 127(1):122–31.

68. Uy GL, Rettig MP, Vey N, et al. Phase 1 cohort expansion of flotetuzumab, a CD123×CD3 Bispecific Dart® protein in patients with relapsed/refractory acute myeloid leukemia (AML). Blood 2018;132(Supplement 1):764, 60 ASH Annual Meeting and Exposition. San Diego, December 1–4, 2018.

69. Chen J, Olsen J, Ford S, et al. A new isoform of interleukin-3 receptor {alpha} with novel differentiation activity and high affinity binding mode. J Biol Chem 2009; 284(9):5763–73.

70. Kovtun Y, Jones GE, Adams S, et al. A CD123-targeting antibody-drug conjugate, IMGN632, designed to eradicate AML while sparing normal bone marrow cells. Blood Adv 2018;2(8):848–58.

71. Sun Q, Woodcock JM, Rapoport A, et al. Monoclonal antibody 7G3 recognizes the N-terminal domain of the human interleukin-3 (IL-3) receptor alpha-chain and functions as a specific IL-3 receptor antagonist. Blood 1996;87(1):83–92.

72. He SZ, Busfield S, Ritchie DS, et al. A phase 1 study of the safety, pharmacokinetics and anti-leukemic activity of the anti-CD123 monoclonal antibody CSL360 in relapsed, refractory or high-risk acute myeloid leukemia. Leuk Lymphoma 2015;56(5):1406–15.

73. Herzog E, Busfield S, Biondo M, et al. Pharmacodynamic activity and preclinical safety of CSL362, a novel humanised, affinity matured monoclonal antibody against human interleukin 3 receptor. Blood 2012;120(21):3598, 54th ASH Annual Meeting and Ezposition. Atlanta, December 8–11, 2012.

74. Busfield SJ, Biondo M, Wond M, et al. CSL362: a monoclonal antibody to human interleukin-3 receptor (CD123), optimized for NK cell-mediated cytotoxicity of AML stem cells. Blood 2012;120(21):3598, 54th ASH Annual Meeting an Exposition. Atlanta, December 8–11, 2012.

75. Busfield SJ, Biondo M, Wong M, et al. Targeting of acute myeloid leukemia in vitro and in vivo with an anti-CD123 mAb engineered for optimal ADCC. Leukemia 2014;28(11):2213–21.

76. Lee EM, Yee D, Busfield SJ, et al. Efficacy of an Fc-modified anti-CD123 antibody (CSL362) combined with chemotherapy in xenograft models of acute myelogenous leukemia in immunodeficient mice. Haematologica 2015;100(7):914–26.

77. Xie LH, Biondo M, Busfield SJ, et al. CD123 target validation and preclinical evaluation of ADCC activity of anti-CD123 antibody CSL362 in combination with NKs from AML patients in remission. Blood Cancer J 2017;7(6):e567.

78. Tettamanti S, Marin V, Pizzitola I, et al. Targeting of acute myeloid leukaemia by cytokine-induced killer cells redirected with a novel CD123-specific chimeric antigen receptor. Br J Haematol 2013;161(3):389–401.

79. Mardiros A, Dos Santos C, McDonald T, et al. T cells expressing CD123-specific chimeric antigen receptors exhibit specific cytolytic effector functions and anti-tumor effects against human acute myeloid leukemia. Blood 2013;122(18): 3138–48.

80. Arcangeli S, Rtiroti MC, Bardelli M, et al. Balance of Anti-CD123 chimeric antigen receptor binding affinity and density for the targeting of acute myeloid leukemia. Mol Ther 2017;25(8):1933–45.

81. Tasian SK, Kenderian SS, Shen F, et al. Optimized depletion of chimeric antigen receptor T cells in murine xenograft models of human acute myeloid leukemia. Blood 2017;129(17):2395–407.

82. Guzman ML, Sugita M, Zong H, et al. Allogeneic Tcrα/β deficient CAR T-cells targeting CD123 prolong overall survival of AML patient-derived xenografts. Blood 2016;128(22):765, 58 ASH Annual Meeting and Exposition. San Diego, December 3–6, 2016.

83. Ruella M, Klichinsky M, Kenderian SS, et al. Overcoming the immunosuppressive tumor microenvironment of Hodgkin lymphoma using chimeric antigen receptor T cells. Cancer Discov 2017;7(10):1154–67.

84. Woll PS, Kjällquist U, Chowdhury O, et al. Myelodysplastic syndromes are propagated by rare and distinct human cancer stem cells in vivo. Cancer Cell 2014; 25(6):794–808.

85. Topp MS, Gölbuget N, Zugmaier G, et al. Phase II trial of the anti-CD19 bispecific T cell-engager blinatumomab shows hematologic and molecular remissions in patients with relapsed or refractory B-precursor acute lymphoblastic leukemia. J Clin Oncol 2014;32(36):4134–40.

86. Maude SL, Frey N, Shaw PA, et al. Chimeric antigen receptor T cells for sustained remissions in leukemia. N Engl J Med 2014;371(16):1507–17.

87. Ruella M, Barrett DM, Kenderian SS, et al. Dual CD19 and CD123 targeting prevents antigen-loss relapses after CD19-directed immunotherapies. J Clin Invest 2016;126(10):3814–26.

88. Aldinucci D, Polleto D, Gloghini A, et al. Expression of functional interleukin-3 receptors on Hodgkin and Reed-Sternberg cells. Am J Pathol 2002;160(2):585–96.

89. Gustafson MP, Lin Y, Maas ML, et al. A method for identification and analysis of non-overlapping myeloid immunophenotypes in humans. PLoS One 2015;10(3): e0121546.

90. Delettre F, Frankel AE, Seilles E, et al. Preclinical studies of SL-401, a targeted therapy directed to the interleukin-3 receptor (IL3-R), in blastic plasmacytoid dendritic cell neoplasm (BPDCN): potent activity in BPDCN cell lines, primary tumor, and in an in vivo model. Blood 2013;122(21):3942, 55 ASH Annual Meeting and Exposition. New Orleans, December 7–10, 2013.

91. Frankel AE, Woo JH, Pemmaraju N, et al. Activity of SL-401, a targeted therapy directed to interleukin-3 receptor, in blastic plasmacytoid dendritic cell neoplasm patients. Blood 2014;124(3):385–92.

92. Pemmaraju N, Lane AA, Sweet KL, et al. Tagraxofusp in blastic plasmacytoid dendritic-cell neoplasm. N Engl J Med 2019;380(17):1628–37.

93. Cai T, Galetto R, Gouble A, et al. Pre-clinical studies of anti-CD123 CAR-T cells for the treatment of blastic plasmacytoid dendritic cell neoplasm (BPDCN). Blood 2016;128(22):4039, 58 ASH Annual Meeting and Exposition. San Diego, December 3–6, 2016.

Tagraxofusp for Blastic Plasmacytoid Dendritic Cell Neoplasm

Danielle Hammond, MD, Naveen Pemmaraju, MD*

KEYWORDS

- BPDCN • Tagraxofusp • CD123 • Interleukin-3 • Diphtheria toxin

KEY POINTS

- Ubiquitous CD123 overexpression is characteristic of BPDCN, an orphan hematologic malignancy. This was the basis for investigating the use of tagraxofusp, a CD123-targeted diphtheria immunotoxin.
- A pilot study and subsequent larger phase I/II trial of tagraxofusp monotherapy in adults with BPDCN demonstrated response rates as high as 90% in frontline-treated patients, including remissions permitting successful bridging to hematopoietic stem cell transplant in 45% of patients in this frontline group.
- The most common treatment-related toxicities are transaminitis and thrombocytopenia. The most serious treatment-related toxicity is capillary leak syndrome.
- Combining tagraxofusp with hypomethylating agents and/or BCL-2 inhibitors are rational next lines of investigation for the treatment of BPDCN.

INTRODUCTION

Progress in the treatment of blastic plasmacytoid dendritic cell neoplasm (BPDCN) has been hampered by the disease's rarity and poorly understood pathogenesis.[1] Although durable remissions can be achieved with hematopoietic stem cell transplantation (HSCT),[2,3] there is no consensus on how to therapeutically bridge patients to transplant or how to treat patients unfit for high-dose chemotherapy. This is reflected by the array of chemotherapy regimens that have historically been used in BPDCN, repurposed from the treatment of more common myeloid and lymphoid malignancies,[4] which is reviewed elsewhere in this issue. Tagraxofusp (DT388IL3; SL-401; Tagraxofusp-ezrs; Elzonris, Stemline Therapeutics) is an intravenously administered CD123-targeted diphtheria toxin (DT) conjugate, which was approved by the Food and Drug Administration (FDA) in December 2018 for the treatment of

Department of Leukemia, The University of Texas MD Anderson Cancer Center, 1515 Holcombe Boulevard, Houston, TX 77030, USA
* Corresponding author.
E-mail address: npemmaraju@mdanderson.org
Twitter: @DanielleHammo20 (D.H.); @doctorpemm (N.P.)

Hematol Oncol Clin N Am 34 (2020) 565–574
https://doi.org/10.1016/j.hoc.2020.01.005
0889-8588/20/© 2020 Elsevier Inc. All rights reserved.

adults and children aged 2 years and older with BPDCN.[5] As a first-in-class approval and the first drug approved for the treatment of BPDCN, tagraxofusp represents a welcome foothold in the burgeoning era of targeted therapy for this rare cancer. The authors review the mechanism of action, preclinical data, and phase I/II clinical trial experience with tagraxofusp in BPDCN. The authors also discuss how the proposed mechanisms of tagraxofusp resistance inform rational combinations for future investigation. Although tagraxofusp is under investigation in several other hematologic malignancies (eg, NCT02270463, NCT02268253, and NCT02661022), its use in those settings is beyond the scope of this review.

LITERATURE REVIEW

A literature review of the MEDLINE database for articles in English using the search terms DT, immunotoxin, interleukin-3/interleukin-3 receptor, tagraxofusp/SL-401/DT388IL3 in conjunction with BPCDN was conducted via PubMed. A total of 183 publications from 1985 through September 2019 were examined. Conference abstracts from the previous decade of the American Society of Hematology, American Society of Clinical Oncology, and European Hematology Association were searched manually. Additional relevant publications were identified by reviewing the references from the selected publications.

MECHANISM OF ACTION

Interleukin-3 (IL-3), which is mainly produced by activated T-lymphocytes, is a pleiotropic cytokine that supports the differentiation of hematopoietic stem cells into myeloid progenitors and serves as a critical aspect of myeloid progenitor survival.[6] CD123 is the alpha subunit of its cognate heterodimeric receptor, IL-3R.[7] Under normal circumstances, CD123 is expressed on plasmacytoid dendritic cells (pDCs),[8] myeloid progenitors,[9] and endothelial cells.[10] Importantly, CD123 expression is absent/low on most hematopoietic stem cells and mature mononuclear cells,[11] suggesting that hematopoiesis would not be unduly impaired by therapies targeting this receptor. In contrast, CD123 is overexpressed on the so-called acute myeloid leukemia (AML) leukemia stem cell population.[12,13] CD123 expression is also enriched to various degrees in myelodysplastic syndromes,[14] chronic myeloid leukemia,[15] Philadelphia-negative myeloproliferative neoplasms,[16] acute lymphoblastic leukemia (ALL),[17] hairy cell leukemia,[18] and even in Hodgkin lymphomas.[19] The translational relevance of CD123 extends to modulation of dendritic cells in the bone marrow milieu: upregulation of IL-3 is thought to mediate a tumor-promoting relationship between the pDCs in the marrow microenvironment and the clonal myeloma cells in multiple myeloma.[20,21] Similar to its healthy cellular counterpart,[8] BPDCN stands out because of its ubiquitous and intense surface CD123 expression.[22] Furthermore, the growth of BPDCN blasts in vitro has been shown to be dependent on IL-3 supplementation.[23] This positions CD123 as a particularly attractive therapeutic target in BPDCN.

Tagraxofusp consists of recombinant human IL-3 fused to a truncated DT. Like the bacterial toxins of *Pseudomonas aeruginosa* and *Vibrio cholerae*, DT induces cellular apoptosis by blocking translation elongation and thus protein synthesis. It does so by catalyzing ADP-ribosylation of the eukaryotic elongation factor 2 protein.[24] Binding of the IL-3 component of tagraxofusp to CD123 triggers a receptor-mediated endocytosis, ultimately releasing the DT catalytic domain into the cytosol where it inactivates protein synthesis.[25] DT fusion proteins have at least 2 mechanistic advantages over traditional cytotoxic agents in the treatment of cancer. By virtue of its interference with protein as opposed to DNA synthesis, a DT fusion protein has shown the ability to kill leukemic cells in the G0 phase.[26] Second, DT is not a known substrate for multidrug resistance drug efflux pumps, such as P-glycoprotein.[27]

PRECLINICAL DEVELOPMENT

Both patient-derived BPDCN blasts and BPDCN cell lines have shown marked sensitivity to tagraxofusp, with femtomolar half-maximal inhibitory concentration values and a clear correlation between CD123 expression and in vitro cytotoxicity.[28] This translated to prolonged survival in a tagraxofusp-treated xenograft mouse model of BPDCN.[29] Moreover, a diphtheria fusion protein demonstrated synergy in combination with cytosine arabinoside in a mouse AML model.[30] A similar finding has recently been reported in an in vitro model of BPDCN.[31] The safety evaluation of tagraxofusp in *Macaca fascicularis* monkeys—which have cross-reactive IL-3 receptors—foreshadowed the subsequent in-human experience in an important respect.[32] One female monkey died of "severe vasculitis of multiple tissues" at a dose of 100 μg/kg. This phenomenon likely represented the primate counterpart of capillary leak syndrome (CLS).

CLINICAL EXPERIENCE IN ADULTS

As reported by Frankel and colleagues,[33] the pilot phase I/II experience with tagraxofusp included 11 adult patients with BPDCN, 4 of whom were treatment-naive. All 11 patients were men with a median age of 68 years. The maximally tolerated dose was greater than 12.5 μg/kg, but 12.5 μg/kg per day was estimated to have the most favorable risk-benefit profile moving forward. Most patients had detectable anti-drug antibodies (ADAs), presumably from diphtheria immunization, which increased on drug exposure. However, neither pretreatment nor posttreatment antibody titers correlated with pharmacokinetics, toxicity, or clinical response. Three of the 11 patients with BPDCN who had an initial response received a second course of tagraxofusp at relapse. Patients received all 5 planned doses 64% of the time (9/14 treatment courses). One patient died of progressive disease after receiving only a single dose of tagraxofusp; there were no treatment-related deaths. Hepatocellular transaminitis and then-called vascular leak syndrome (VLS) were the 2 most notable toxicities, both which were dose-dependent. Although most patients developed some degree of transaminitis, it was rapidly reversible. Nonetheless, transaminitis resulted in treatment discontinuation in 2 patients. VLS presented as a constellation of hypoalbuminemia ± edema, rapid weight gain, hypotension, hypoxia, and acute kidney injury. Therefore, treatment was only permitted if the serum albumin was ≥3 g/dL. If their serum albumin decreased below 3 g/dL on infusion days or in the immediate posttreatment period, patients could receive 25 g of intravenous albumin daily. Infusion-related reactions (eg, fever and chills) were common but easily managed. Thrombocytopenia was frequent, whereas the other peripheral blood counts were spared, hypothesized to be due to the relative dependence of megakaryopoiesis on IL-3.[34] Although the clinical implications of targeting healthy pDCs is unclear, there was no signal of infectious complications. Seventy-eight percent (7 out of 9 evaluable patients) had either a complete response ([CR], 5 patients) or partial response ([PR], 2 patients) after just a single course of tagraxofusp. CR was defined as normalization of peripheral blood counts and the bone marrow, absence of disease on PET/CT imaging, normal liver and spleen size without nodules, and absence of skin involvement documented by examination and biopsy of previously affected areas. Responses occurred irrespective of the disease sites involved. However, the median response duration was limited: 5 months (range, 1–20+ months).

Those encouraging results were the basis of the subsequent largest prospective study ever conducted in patients with BPDCN (NCT02113982).[35] It was a multicenter, nonrandomized, open-label, multicohort study of adult patients with both treatment-naive and relapsed/refractory BPDCN. Patients with AML were also permitted to participate in the first 2 phases of the study; report of their outcomes is limited.[36] There were 2 exclusion criteria of note. The first was known central nervous system (CNS) disease. Although symptomatic CNS involvement is common at relapse,[37] 1 series identified clinically silent CNS disease on baseline lumbar punctures at initial diagnosis in 6/10 consecutive patients with BPDCN.[38] Lumbar punctures to assess for such occult CNS disease were not performed in this study. The second was the requirement for a baseline serum albumin ≥3.2 g/dL, similar to the pilot study, attentive to the risk of CLS. Given the previous lack of consensus response criteria for BPDCN, the investigators developed a comprehensive set of criteria reflecting the most commonly involved sites of disease (in order of decreasing frequency: skin, bone marrow, lymph nodes, and viscera). As used in cutaneous T cell lymphomas, the Modified Severity Weighted Assessment Tool was applied to quantify the extent of cutaneous involvement.[39] Reflecting the unusual predilection of BPDCN for the skin, response criteria included the novel outcome of CR with minimal residual cutaneous abnormality (CRc). It is defined as clinical CR of all non-skin disease compartments and marked clearance of all previous skin lesions, but in which there is residual hyperpigmentation or microscopic residual disease on biopsy (or no biopsy performed). Importantly, CRc reflected the lack of active skin disease and was validated as a measure of clinical benefit. Forty-seven adult patients with BPDCN were enrolled over a 4-year period, 32 who were treatment-naive and 15 who had received previous therapy. In the latter group, 6 had received 2 or more previous lines of therapy; the treatment regimens were not specified. The study had 4 development phases; both treatment-naive and previously treated patients were enrolled in the first 2 dose escalation and expansion phases, respectively. Only treatment-naive patients were permitted in the "pivotal" third stage; stage 4 was a continued access phase. The median age was 68 years (range, 22–84 years), and there was a predominance of men in line with historical expectations (81%). Almost all patients had skin involvement and 47% had bone marrow involvement. No baseline immunohistochemical, cytogenetic, or mutation data were reported. Three patients in the dose escalation phase who received tagraxofusp at the 7-μg/kg dose were included in the safety but not efficacy analysis. All other patients received 12 μg/kg/day and were included in the efficacy analysis. The dosing schedule was days 1 to 5 (with a 10-day treatment window to allow for dose delays) on a 21-day cycle. Cycles could be repeated until disease progression or unacceptable adverse effects. Tagraxofusp was generally given in the inpatient setting (with the option for outpatient administration of subsequent cycles at the discretion of the treating physician) with close monitoring for CLS, including daily serum albumin, blood pressure, and body weight measurements. Supplemental intravenous albumin was given on treatment days per protocol-specified CLS management guidelines that were optimized during the first stage of the trial. The primary endpoint was a composite of CR and CRc. Of the 29 treatment-naive patients receiving the 12-μg/kg dose, the CR plus CRc rate was 72% (95% CI, 53%–87%). The overall response rate ([ORR], PR, or better) was 90% with a median time to response of 43 days (95% CI, 14–131). After a median follow-up of 19 months, the median duration of CR plus CRc was not reached in this group. After a median follow-up of 25 months, the median overall survival (OS) had not been reached with a survival probability of 52% at 2 years. Critically, 13 (45%) of the treatment-naive patients went on to receive a consolidative HSCT after a response to tagraxofusp (10 allogeneic, 3 autologous). One of these patients was bridged to transplant while in PR as opposed to CR/CRc, yet they had an excellent duration of response (903+ days) and OS (919+ days). In the 15 previously treated patients, the ORR was 67% with a median time to response of 24 days (range, 17–48 days). In the 10 responders, 2 had a CR/CRc, 3 had a CR with incomplete count recovery (CRi), and 5 had a PR. The presence of CRi in this group likely reflects the cumulative myelosuppressive effect of previous lines of therapy. In previously treated patients, the median duration of response was 2.8 months and the median survival was 8.5 months. One patient in this group was successfully bridged to an allogeneic HSCT while in CRc. Similar to the pilot experience, the most common treatment-related adverse events were hepatocellular transaminitis, isolated thrombocytopenia, and CLS or its related manifestations (eg, hypoalbuminemia, hypotension). There was a comparable incidence of ≥ grade 3 adverse events in treatment-naive (87%) versus previously treated (78%) patients, most of these being asymptomatic, reversible increases in the transaminases. Thrombocytopenia to any degree was seen in 40% of patients. CLS occurred in 18% of patients, with 6 out of 8 cases being moderate (grade 2) in severity. However, the 2 remaining cases resulted in death, 1 occurring at the 7-μg/kg dose and the other occurring at the 12-μg/kg dose. The first death occurred before implementing additional safety measures reflected in the updated CLS management guidelines. All but 1 case of CLS occurred during the first cycle of therapy, with a median time to onset of 5 days (range, 4–51 days) and median duration of 4 days (range, 3–19 days). All episodes were treated with intravenous albumin. Additional measures included withholding additional doses until resolution, careful management of volume status (eg, crystalloids if hypotensive or increased creatinine, diuretics if fluid-overloaded), and corticosteroids. Importantly, an initial decrease in serum albumin was the most reliable predictor of developing CLS. As in the pilot trial, most patients had pre-existing ADAs, presumably from diphtheria immunization.[40] Including participating patients with either BPDCN or AML, 21% had neutralizing antibodies.

PEDIATRIC BLASTIC PLASMACYTOID DENDRITIC CELL NEOPLASM: CLINICAL EXPERIENCE IN CHILDREN

Although several studies put the median age at diagnosis of BPDCN closer to 70 years,[37,41] a recent Surveillance Epidemiology and End Results database review conducted in the United States found that the median age at diagnosis was approximately 53 years.[42] This reflected a bimodal age distribution with the first peak in those younger than 20 years. In 2018, Sun and colleagues[43] reported the first pediatric experience with compassionate use tagraxofusp in 3 patients treated at The City of Hope National Medical Center. The first patient was a 10-year-old girl who received 2 cycles of tagraxofusp in third salvage after 3 lines of chemotherapy, including 1 line of decitabine. Although she previously had CNS disease, her cerebrospinal fluid was negative on starting tagraxofusp. She had stable disease after the first course of therapy; however, there was disease progression during the second course and she died 5 months later after another line of salvage chemotherapy. She had infusion-type reactions with both the first (flushing, fever) and second (tachycardia, hypoxia) courses, respectively. The second patient was a 12-year-old girl who received tagraxofusp frontline given her family's desire to avoid cytotoxic chemotherapy. She received 5 cycles without any major adverse events. After the first 2 cycles, there was a marked reduction in the size of her index soft tissue mass. However, after cycles 4 and 5, there was subsequent disease progression. She reached a CR with salvage hyper-CVAD and remained in remission 1 year after unrelated cord blood allogeneic HSCT. The third patient was a 15-year-old girl who received 2 cycles of tagraxofusp in third salvage for chemo-refractory disease. She had a PR after the first cycle due to a marked improvement in disease involvement in the lungs and marrow. The second course was delayed for nonmedical reasons, and she had secondary disease progression (new skin lesions and adenopathy). Again, there was improvement and/or resolution of all previous disease sites after receiving the second cycle. However, she developed additional extramedullary disease (breast, orbital) that was stable after a third cycle but progressed after the forth cycle. She died from progressive disease a few months thereafter. The fifth dose of the first and second cycles were both held due to early markers of CLS (hypoalbuminemia and rapid weight gain). The patient with the best outcome received tagraxofusp in the frontline setting and was the only patient to be subsequently bridged to an HSCT. However, additional ALL-type chemotherapy was required to achieve a pretransplant remission. Sun and colleagues also observed that, in 2 patients, CD123 expression was preserved at the time of disease progression on tagraxofusp, which is relevant to the last section of this review. These data, although from only a handful of patients, was the basis of the FDA approval, including children 2 years and older.

CONTEXT FOR THE EARLY CLINICAL EXPERIENCE

In a review of a cohort of patients with BPDCN treated at academic centers before the availability of tagraxofusp, only 55% received intensive induction-type chemotherapy.[4] Receiving intensive chemotherapy as opposed to less-intensive regimens had a striking 2-year progression-free survival benefit (45% vs 11%; $P = .034$). This was driven in large part by the ability to undergo subsequent consolidative allogeneic or autologous HSCT. Therefore, it is even more notable that 45% of patients in the treatment-naive cohort in the pivotal phase I/II tagraxofusp trial were successfully bridged to transplant using immunotoxin monotherapy. The flipside being that without a consolidative strategy, responses to tagraxofusp seem to be limited, especially in previously treated patients, owing to the inherently aggressive nature of BPDCN.

In contrast to the adult experience with tagraxofusp, none of the 3 reported pediatric cases achieved a CR and responses were shorter lived. This may reflect instructive differences in the biology of BPDCN in children versus adults.[44,45] However, this may alternatively represent pharmacokinetic or other metabolic differences. A comprehensive review of BPDCN in children is provided elsewhere in this issue.

Patients with known CNS disease were excluded from the study by Pemmaraju and colleagues, and no concurrent intrathecal prophylaxis was administered. Despite this, there were no cases of overt CNS disease appearing while on tagraxofusp. Whether tagraxofusp can penetrate the blood-brain barrier and is active in BPDCN and other CD123-expressing malignancies in the CNS compartment is unknown: this will be of interest for future investigation.

Dose-limiting CLS has been reported with other immunotoxins, including a DT and interleukin-2 fusion protein evaluated in the treatment of cutaneous T-cell lymphomas.[46,47] The purported mechanism is direct endothelial toxicity and drug-protein aggregates that interact with the endothelium, disrupting the tight junctions.[48] Interestingly, investigators were able to reduce vascular leak in a mouse model of melanoma treated with a DT fusion protein by engineering a single amino acid substitution in a vascular leak-inducing motif in the DT sequence.[49] From a clinical perspective, it is essential that patients are selected carefully for tagraxofusp therapy. They should have a normal pretreatment cardiac function and serum albumin level, given the rapid intravascular volume shifts characteristic of CLS.

Although immunization-related ADAs have been demonstrated, their clinical significance seems to be minimal in the use of tagraxofusp for BPDCN. This is likely because only a minority of the antibodies are neutralizing and that BPDCN blasts are exquisitely sensitive to the drug.

NEXT STEPS: RATIONAL COMBINATION THERAPY

Togami and colleagues[31] provided several insights into mechanisms of tagraxofusp resistance, identifying hypomethylating agents and antiapoptotic proteins as ideal partner agents to overcome and/or prevent tagraxofusp failure. Using patient-derived and in vitro AML and BPDCN cell lines, they demonstrated that drug resistance was not associated with CD123 downregulation or failure to traffic the fusion protein. Rather, it originated from resistance to the ADP-ribosylation mechanism central to DT cytotoxicity. Eukaryotic elongation factor 2, the protein target of DT, contains a posttranslationally modified histidine residue called diphthamide. Diphthamide biosynthesis involves a multistep enzymatically mediated pathway.[50] They demonstrated that tagraxofusp resistance was mediated by DNA CpG methylation of the *DPH1* locus, leading to reduced expression of a key diphthamide pathway enzyme. Notably, this resistance could be overcome by the addition of azacitidine, a hypomethylating agent. The second important finding was that, at the time of tagraxofusp resistance, AML and BPDCN cells actually had increased apoptotic priming, supporting the future study of BCL-2 inhibitors and other antiapoptotic proteins in combination with tagraxofusp and/or other agents.[51–53] The first finding was the impetus for the actively recruiting phase 1 trial of tagraxofusp and azacitidine in patients with AML or high-risk MDS (NCT03113643). At the time of writing this review, no similar trial of tagraxofusp combination therapy is open for patients with BPDCN. Finally, Togami and colleagues also developed a flow cytometry-based drug-dependent ADP-ribosylation assay that, if validated, could serve to identify patients most likely to respond to tagraxofusp-based regimens.

"If you don't know where you've come from, you don't know where you're going." Taylor and colleagues recently presented a review of clinical characteristics, pretransplant treatment regimens, and outcomes of 59 adult patients with BPDCN treated at 3 US referral cancer centers in the pre-tagraxofusp era.[4] This cohort will serve as an invaluable historical benchmark with which to compare outcomes with tagraxofusp and other novel regimens moving forward.

DISCLOSURE

D. Hammond has nothing to disclose. N. Pemmaraju declares the following: Consulting/honorarium from Celgene, Stemline, Incyte Corporation, Novartis, MustangBio, Roche Diagnostics, and LFB. Research funding/clinical trials support from Stemline, Novartis, Abbvie, Samus, Cellectis, Plexxikon, Daiichi-Sankyo, Affymetrix, and Sager-Strong Foundation. This research is supported in part by the MD Anderson Cancer Center support grant P30 CA016672.

REFERENCES

1. Pemmaraju N, Utengen A, Gupta V, et al. Analysis of first-year twitter metrics of a rare disease community for blastic plasmacytoid dendritic cell neoplasm (BPDCN) on social media: #BPDCN. Curr Hematol Malig Rep 2017;12(6):592–7.
2. Aoki T, Suzuki R, Kuwatsuka Y, et al. Long-term survival following autologous and allogeneic stem cell transplantation for blastic plasmacytoid dendritic cell neoplasm. Blood 2015;125(23):3559–62.

3. Kharfan-Dabaja MA, Reljic T, Murthy HS, et al. Allogeneic hematopoietic cell transplantation is an effective treatment for blastic plasmacytoid dendritic cell neoplasm in first complete remission: systematic review and meta-analysis. Clin Lymphoma Myeloma Leuk 2018;18(11):703–9.e1.

4. Taylor J, Haddadin M, Upadhyay VA, et al. Multicenter analysis of outcomes in blastic plasmacytoid dendritic cell neoplasm offers a pretargeted therapy benchmark. Blood 2019;134(8):678–87.

5. Stemline Therapeutics. ELZONRIS (tagraxofusp-erzs): highlights of prescribing information. 2018. Available at: https://www.accessdata.fda.gov/drugsatfda_docs/label/2018/761116s000lbl.pdf. Accessed: August 21, 2019.

6. Suda T, Suda J, Ogawa M, et al. Permissive role of interleukin 3 (IL-3) in proliferation and differentiation of multipotential hemopoietic progenitors in culture. J Cell Physiol 1985;124(2):182–90.

7. Feuring-Buske M, Frankel AE, Alexander RL, et al. A diphtheria toxin-interleukin 3 fusion protein is cytotoxic to primitive acute myeloid leukemia progenitors but spares normal progenitors. Cancer Res 2002;62(6):1730–6.

8. MacDonald KP, Munster DJ, Clark GJ, et al. Characterization of human blood dendritic cell subsets. Blood 2002;100(13):4512–20.

9. Testa U, Fossati C, Samoggia P, et al. Expression of growth factor receptors in unilineage differentiation culture of purified hematopoietic progenitors. Blood 1996;88(9):3391–406.

10. Brizzi MF, Garbarino G, Rossi PR, et al. Interleukin 3 stimulates proliferation and triggers endothelial-leukocyte adhesion molecule 1 gene activation of human endothelial cells. J Clin Invest 1993;91(6):2887–92.

11. Jin L, Lee EM, Ramshaw HS, et al. Monoclonal antibody-mediated targeting of CD123, IL-3 receptor alpha chain, eliminates human acute myeloid leukemic stem cells. Cell Stem Cell 2009;5(1):31–42.

12. Jordan CT, Upchurch D, Szilvassy SJ, et al. The interleukin-3 receptor alpha chain is a unique marker for human acute myelogenous leukemia stem cells. Leukemia 2000;14(10):1777–84.

13. Testa U, Riccioni R, Diverio D, et al. Interleukin-3 receptor in acute leukemia. Leukemia 2004;18(2):219–26.

14. Li LJ, Tao JL, Fu R, et al. Increased CD34+CD38-CD123+ cells in myelodysplastic syndrome displaying malignant features similar to those in AML. Int J Hematol 2014;100(1):60–9.

15. Nievergall E, Ramshaw HS, Yong AS, et al. Monoclonal antibody targeting of IL-3 receptor α with CSL362 effectively depletes CML progenitor and stem cells. Blood 2014;123(8):1218–28.

16. Lasho T, Finke C, Kimlinger TK, et al. Expression of CD123 (IL-3R-alpha), a therapeutic target of SL-401, on myeloproliferative neoplasms. Blood 2014;124(21):5577.

17. Djokic M, Björklund E, Blennow E, et al. Overexpression of CD123 correlates with the hyperdiploid genotype in acute lymphoblastic leukemia. Haematologica 2009;94(7):1016–9.

18. Shao H, Calvo KR, Grönborg M, et al. Distinguishing hairy cell leukemia variant from hairy cell leukemia: development and validation of diagnostic criteria. Leuk Res 2013;37(4):401–9.

19. Aldinucci D, Poletto D, Gloghini A, et al. Expression of functional interleukin-3 receptors on Hodgkin and Reed-Sternberg cells. Am J Pathol 2002;160(2):585–96.

20. Leone P, Berardi S, Frassanito MA, et al. Dendritic cells accumulate in the bone marrow of myeloma patients where they protect tumor plasma cells from CD8+ T-cell killing. Blood 2015;126(12):1443–51.

21. Ray A, Das DS, Song Y, et al. A novel agent SL-401 induces anti-myeloma activity by targeting plasmacytoid dendritic cells, osteoclastogenesis and cancer stem-like cells. Leukemia 2017;31(12):2652–60.

22. Garnache-Ottou F, Feuillard J, Ferrand C, et al. Extended diagnostic criteria for plasmacytoid dendritic cell leukaemia. Br J Haematol 2009;145(5):624–36.

23. Chaperot L, Bendriss N, Manches O, et al. Identification of a leukemic counterpart of the plasmacytoid dendritic cells. Blood 2001;97(10):3210–7.

24. Cohen MS, Chang P. Insights into the biogenesis, function, and regulation of ADP-ribosylation. Nat Chem Biol 2018;14:236.

25. FitzGerald DJ. Targeted diphtheria toxin to treat BPDCN. Blood 2014;124(3): 310–2.

26. Jedema I, Barge RM, Frankel AE, et al. Acute myeloid leukemia cells in G0 phase of the cell cycle that are unresponsive to conventional chemotherapy are sensitive to treatment with granulocyte-macrophage colony-stimulating factor/diphtheria toxin fusion proteins. Exp Hematol 2004;32(2):188–94.

27. Frankel AE, Hall PD, McLain C, et al. Cell-specific modulation of drug resistance in acute myeloid leukemic blasts by diphtheria fusion toxin, DT388-GMCSF. Bioconjug Chem 1998;9(4):490–6.

28. Angelot-Delettre F, Roggy A, Frankel AE, et al. In vivo and in vitro sensitivity of blastic plasmacytoid dendritic cell neoplasm to SL-401, an interleukin-3 receptor targeted biologic agent. Haematologica 2015;100(2):223–30.

29. Frankel AE, Seilles E, Biichle S, et al. Preclinical studies of SL-401, a targeted therapy directed to the interleukin-3 receptor (IL3-R), in blastic plasmacytoid dendritic cell neoplasm (BPDCN): potent activity In BPDCN cell lines, primary tumor, and in an in vivo model. Blood 2013;122(21):3942.

30. Hogge DE, Feuring-Buske M, Gerhard B, et al. The efficacy of diphtheria-growth factor fusion proteins is enhanced by co-administration of cytosine arabinoside in an immunodeficient mouse model of human acute myeloid leukemia. Leuk Res 2004;28(11):1221–6.

31. Togami K, Pastika T, Stephansky J, et al. DNA methyltransferase inhibition overcomes diphthamide pathway deficiencies underlying CD123-targeted treatment resistance. J Clin Invest 2019;129(11):5005–19.

32. Cohen KA, Liu TF, Cline JM, et al. Safety evaluation of DT388IL3, a diphtheria toxin/interleukin 3 fusion protein, in the cynomolgus monkey. Cancer Immunol Immunother 2005;54(8):799–806.

33. Frankel AE, Woo JH, Ahn C, et al. Activity of SL-401, a targeted therapy directed to interleukin-3 receptor, in blastic plasmacytoid dendritic cell neoplasm patients. Blood 2014;124(3):385–92.

34. Chen TW, Hwang SM, Chu IM, et al. Characterization and transplantation of induced megakaryocytes from hematopoietic stem cells for rapid platelet recovery by a two-step serum-free procedure. Exp Hematol 2009;37(11):1330–9.e5.

35. Pemmaraju N, Lane AA, Sweet KL, et al. Tagraxofusp in blastic plasmacytoid dendritic-cell neoplasm. N Engl J Med 2019;380(17):1628–37.

36. Sweet KL, Pemmaraju N, Lane AA, et al. Lead-in stage results of a pivotal trial of SL-401, an interleukin-3 receptor (IL-3R) targeting biologic, in patients with blastic plasmacytoid dendritic cell neoplasm (BPDCN) or acute myeloid leukemia (AML). Blood 2015;126(23):3795.

37. Pagano L, Valentini CG, Pulsoni A, et al. Blastic plasmacytoid dendritic cell neoplasm with leukemic presentation: an Italian multicenter study. Haematologica 2013;98(2):239–46.

38. Martín-Martín L, Almeida J, Pomares H, et al. Blastic plasmacytoid dendritic cell neoplasm frequently shows occult central nervous system involvement at diagnosis and benefits from intrathecal therapy. Oncotarget 2016;7(9):10174–81.
39. Olsen EA, Whittaker S, Kim YH, et al. Clinical end points and response criteria in mycosis fungoides and Sézary syndrome: a consensus statement of the International Society for Cutaneous Lymphomas, the United States Cutaneous Lymphoma Consortium, and the Cutaneous Lymphoma Task Force of the European Organisation for Research and Treatment of Cancer. J Clin Oncol 2011;29(18):2598–607.
40. Pazdur R, Farrell A, Przepiorka D. FDA summary review of application number 761116Orig1s000. 2018. Available at: https://www.accessdata.fda.gov/drugsatfda_docs/nda/2018/761116Orig1s000SumR.pdf. Accessed: September 3, 2019.
41. Pemmaraju N. Blastic plasmacytoid dendritic cell neoplasm. Clin Adv Hematol Oncol 2016;14(4):220–2.
42. Guru Murthy GS, Pemmaraju N, Atallah E. Epidemiology and survival of blastic plasmacytoid dendritic cell neoplasm. Leuk Res 2018;73:21–3.
43. Sun W, Liu H, Kim Y, et al. First pediatric experience of SL-401, a CD123-targeted therapy, in patients with blastic plasmacytoid dendritic cell neoplasm: report of three cases. J Hematol Oncol 2018;11(1):61.
44. Nguyen CM, Stuart L, Skupsky H, et al. Blastic plasmacytoid dendritic cell neoplasm in the pediatric population: a case series and review of the literature. Am J Dermatopathol 2015;37(12):924–8.
45. Sakashita K, Saito S, Yanagisawa R, et al. Usefulness of allogeneic hematopoietic stem cell transplantation in first complete remission for pediatric blastic plasmacytoid dendritic cell neoplasm with skin involvement: a case report and review of literature. Pediatr Blood Cancer 2013;60(11):E140–2.
46. Olsen E, Duvic M, Frankel A, et al. Pivotal phase III trial of two dose levels of denileukin diftitox for the treatment of cutaneous T-cell lymphoma. J Clin Oncol 2001;19(2):376–88.
47. Talpur R, Duvic M. Pilot study of denileukin diftitox alternate dosing regimen in patients with cutaneous peripheral T-cell lymphomas. Clin Lymphoma Myeloma Leuk 2012;12(3):180–5.
48. Lindstrom AL, Erlandsen SL, Kersey JH, et al. An in vitro model for toxin-mediated vascular leak syndrome: ricin toxin a chain increases the permeability of human endothelial cell monolayers. Blood 1997;90(6):2323–34.
49. Cheung LS, Fu J, Kumar P, et al. Second-generation IL-2 receptor-targeted diphtheria fusion toxin exhibits antitumor activity and synergy with anti-PD-1 in melanoma. Proc Natl Acad Sci U S A 2019;116(8):3100–5.
50. Su X, Lin Z, Lin H. The biosynthesis and biological function of diphthamide. Crit Rev Biochem Mol Biol 2013;48(6):515–21.
51. DiNardo CD, Rausch CR, Benton C, et al. Clinical experience with the BCL2-inhibitor venetoclax in combination therapy for relapsed and refractory acute myeloid leukemia and related myeloid malignancies. Am J Hematol 2018;93(3):401–7.
52. Montero J, Stephansky J, Cai T, et al. Blastic plasmacytoid dendritic cell neoplasm is dependent on BCL2 and sensitive to venetoclax. Cancer Discov 2017;7(2):156–64.
53. Pemmaraju N, Konopleva M, Lane AA. More on blastic plasmacytoid dendritic-cell neoplasms. N Engl J Med 2019;380(7):695–6.

Immunotherapies Targeting CD123 for Blastic Plasmacytoid Dendritic Cell Neoplasm

Tongyuan Xue, MD[a,b,c,d], L. Elizabeth Budde, MD, PhD[a,c,d],*

KEYWORDS

- Immunotherapies • CD123 • BPDCN • AML • CAR T • ADC • BsAb

KEY POINTS

- CD123 is overexpressed on both acute myeloid leukemia (AML) and BPDCN in comparison with normal hematopoietic stem cells, suggesting CD123 as an attractive immunotherapeutic target.
- Multiple phase 1 clinical trials targeting CD123 using chimeric antigen receptor T cell immunotherapies are under active development for patients with relapsed and/or refractory (r/r) AML and BPDCN.
- Other immunotherapeutic approaches targeting CD123, including antibody-drug conjugate and bispecific antibody, are currently being explored for the treatment of AML and BPDCN.

INTRODUCTION: BLASTIC PLASMACYTOID DENDRITIC CELL NEOPLASM AND CD123

Blastic plasmacytoid dendritic cell neoplasm (BPDCN) is a rare and highly aggressive myeloid malignancy derived from the precursors of plasmacytoid dendritic cells that is difficult to diagnose,.[1–3] In 2008, the World Health Organization (WHO) defined the term BPDCN, categorizing this cancer under AML and related neoplasms.[4] In 2016, BPDCN was redesignated by WHO as its own entity under the category of myeloid malignancies.[5] Approximately 80% to 90% of BPDCN patients present with skin

Grant Support: This review article is supported by the Damon Runyon Cancer Research Foundation.
a Department of Hematology & Hematology Cell Transplantation, City of Hope, 1500 East Duarte Road, Duarte, CA 91010, USA; b Department of Molecular Medicine, Beckman Research Institute, City of Hope, 1500 East Duarte Road, Duarte, CA 91010, USA; c T Cell Therapeutics Research Laboratory, Beckman Research Institute, City of Hope, 1500 East Duarte Road, Duarte, CA 91010, USA; d Irell & Manella Graduate School of Biological Sciences, Beckman Research Institute, City of Hope, 1500 East Duarte Road, Duarte, CA 91010, USA
* Corresponding author. Department of Hematology & Hematology Cell Transplantation, City of Hope, 1500 East Duarte Road, Duarte, CA 91010.
E-mail address: ebudde@coh.org

Hematol Oncol Clin N Am 34 (2020) 575–587
https://doi.org/10.1016/j.hoc.2020.01.006
0889-8588/20/© 2020 Elsevier Inc. All rights reserved.

hemonc.theclinics.com

lesions. Although initially indolent, these lesions rapidly progress to leukemic dissemination that involves bone marrow and/or peripheral blood.[6–10] This dissemination may also manifest with extramedullary organ involvement, including lymph nodes, spleen, liver, and to a certain extent the central nervous system.[2,11–14] BPDCN can present at any age but is more common in elderly patients (mid-to-late sixties).[15–17] There is no known ethnic predisposition for developing BPDCN. However, BPDCN is more commonly diagnosed in males, with a 3:1 male-to-female ratio.[15]

BPDCN has been reported to coincide with chronic myelomonocytic leukemia and myelodysplastic syndrome (MDS). In addition, 15% to 20% of BPDCN eventually transform into AML.[15,18–21] Thus, to distinguish BPDCN from the aforementioned malignancies, diagnosis of BPDCN depends on immunophenotypic criteria based on flow cytometry and immunohistochemistry (IHC) analyses. Specifically, BPDCN is positive for CD123, CD4, CD56, and T cell leukemia/lymphoma 1 and negative for myeloperoxidase and lysozyme.[1,3,22] Given its low incidence and poor prognosis, there is no standard therapy.[21,23,24] Allogenic hematopoietic cell transplantation (allo-HCT) during the first complete remission (CR) can achieve durable regression.[25,26] However, relapse occurs in 30% to 40% of patients who achieve CR[1] and the prognosis at relapse is extremely poor.[27] Taken together, there is an urgent need for novel targeted therapies to improve the treatment of BPDCN.

CD123, also known as interleukin-3 receptor α (IL-3Rα), is a type I transmembrane glycoprotein. CD123 forms dimers with interleukin-3 receptor β (IL-3Rβ), CD131, and is involved in IL-3 signaling. CD123 is highly expressed in AML and nearly all BPDCN cases.[28–30] Jordan and colleagues[31] were the first group to demonstrate that CD123 is strongly expressed on AML leukemic blasts and leukemic stem cells (LSCs, 98 ± 2%) whereas being restricted to <1% on normal hematopoietic stem cells (HSCs). These findings identify that CD123 is a potential therapeutic target for patients with CD123+ hematologic malignancies, including AML and BPDCN.[1,32] Moreover, there is evidence to suggest that overexpression of CD123 correlates with differential sensitivity to therapies and blast proliferation. For instance, Testa and colleagues[33] reported that 70% of patients with AML who had high CD123 expression achieved CR following intensive induction chemotherapy. Chaperot and colleagues[34] proved that BPDCN primary blasts required IL-3 supplementation for in vitro growth and survival. Furthermore, increased levels of CD123 expression were identified in patients with MDS, chronic myeloid leukemia (CML), and aggressive lymphomas.[35–37] Based on these findings, several groups initiated the development of CD123-targeted therapies using multiple immune-based strategies (**Fig. 1**), and have shown promising antileukemic responses in the preclinical setting.[37–39] Several CD123-targeted immunotherapies are currently being tested in clinical trials.[32,40–43] Overall, CD123 has emerged as an attractive immunotherapeutic target for the treatment of CD123+ hematologic malignancies, particularly BPDCN and AML. This review provides an overview of novel immunotherapies that target CD123, including chimeric antigen receptor (CAR) T cells, recombinant fusion protein, antibody-drug conjugate (ADC), and bispecific antibody (BsAb) (**Table 1**).

CD123 CHIMERIC ANTIGEN RECEPTOR T CELL IMMUNOTHERAPY

Distinct from T cell receptor (TCR)-based immunotherapies and conventional chemotherapies, CAR T cell immunotherapy functions in a major histocompatibility complex-independent manner and can confer long-term immunity.[44,45] Recently, CD19CAR T cell therapies have achieved major breakthroughs for treating patients with B cell malignancies, which led to the Food and Drug Administration (FDA) approval of 2

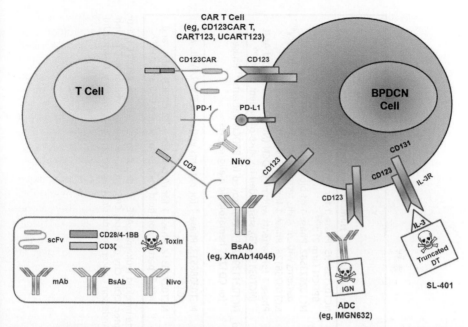

Fig. 1. CD123-targeted immunotherapies for BPDCN treatment. ADC, antibody-drug conjugate; BPDCN, blastic plasmacytoid dendritic cell neoplasm; BsAb, bispecific antibody; CAR, chimeric antigen receptor; CART123, University of Pennsylvania's CD123-targeted CAR T; CD123CAR T, City of Hope's CD123-targeted CAR T; CD28/4-1BB, costimulatory domain; CD3ζ, signaling domain; DT, diphtheria toxin; IGN, indolinobenzodiazepine pseudodimer; IL-3R, IL-3 receptor where CD123 (IL-3Rα) forms dimers with CD131 (IL-3Rβ); mAb, monoclonal antibody; Nivo, nivolumab; PD-1, programmed death-1; PD-L1, programmed death-ligand 1; scFv, single-chain variable fragment; UCART123, MD Anderson Cancer Center/Cellectis' CD123-targeted CAR T.

cellular products for patients with B cell acute lymphoblastic leukemia (B-ALL) and diffuse large B cell lymphoma.[46,47] However, novel and effective immunotherapies for patients with myeloid malignancies, particularly BPDCN and AML, remain an urgent unmet need.

The authors and others have demonstrated the efficacy of CD123CAR T cells against BPDCN and AML in preclinical settings.[48–50] The authors' CD123CAR consists of an anti-CD123 single-chain variable fragment (scFv), an optimized immunoglobulin G_4 hinge domain that reduces Fc receptor binding, a CD28 costimulatory domain, an intracellular CD3ζ signaling domain, and a truncated epidermal growth factor receptor marker for CAR selection, tracking, and potential elimination by cetuximab.[51] The authors have demonstrated that CD123CAR T cells potently kill the human AML KG-1a cell line both in vitro and in vivo. Moreover, when expressed on AML patient-derived T cells, CD123CAR redirects T cell cytotoxicity against autologous blasts. Importantly, colony formation of normal progenitors was not compromised when cord blood–derived CD34⁺ cells were treated with CD123CAR T cells,[48] demonstrating that the CD123CAR T cells did not target normal CD34⁺ progenitor cells. Gill and colleagues[49] generated T cells expressing a second-generation CAR targeting CD123 with a 4-1BB costimulatory domain (CART123). Using a patient-derived xenograft (PDX) model of primary AML, they observed potent antileukemic activity in vivo. However, CART123 cells also disrupted normal myelopoiesis in the PDX model, indicating a

Table 1
Immunotherapies targeting CD123 for BPDCN

Immunotherapy	Product	Developer	Characteristics	ClinicalTrials.gov Number and Stage of Development
CAR T Cell	CD123CAR T	COH	Lentiviral delivery	NCT02159495. Phase 1 for patients with r/r AML (arm 1) and BPDCN (arm 2)[32,53]
	CART123	Upenn	mRNA delivery	NCT02623582. Phase 1 of biodegradable CART123 cells for patients with r/r AML, terminated owing to lack of efficacy[40]
	CART123	Upenn	Lentiviral delivery	NCT03766126. Phase 1 for patients with r/r AML
	UCART123	MDACC/Cellectis	TALEN technology	Phase 1 for patients with r/r BPDCN (NCT03203369) and AML (NCT03190278), suspended because of patient death[56]
Recombinant fusion protein	SL-401, (tagraxofusp, Elzonris)	Stemline Therapeutics	IL-3 fused to a truncated DT payload	NCT02113982. FDA-approved for BPDCN patients.[41] Phase 1/2 for CD123+ hematologic malignancies
ADC	IMGN632	ImmunoGen	Anti-CD123 mAb conjugated to DNA-alkylating payload	NCT03386513. Phase 1 for patients with r/r BPDCN, AML, and ALL[42]
BsAb	XmAb14045	Xencor	Bispecific CD123 × CD3 antibody	NCT02730312. Phase 1 for r/r patients with BPDCN, AML, and ALL,[43] partially on hold because of severe CRS and APE[65]

Abbreviations: ADC, antibody-drug conjugate; ALL, acute lymphoblastic leukemia; AML, acute myeloid leukemia; APE, acute pulmonary edema; BPDCN, blastic plasmacytoid dendritic cell neoplasm; BsAb, bispecific antibody; CAR, chimeric antigen receptor; COH, City of Hope; CRS, cytokine release syndrome; DT, diphtheria toxin; FDA, Food and Drug Administration; mAb, monoclonal antibody; MDACC, MD Anderson Cancer Center; r/r, relapsed and/or refractory; Upenn, University of Pennsylvania.

potentially problematic myeloablative effect. Cai and colleagues[50] manufactured a CD123-targeting allogeneic T cell product (UCART123) consisting of T cells from healthy donors engineered to express a CD123CAR (anti-CD123 scFv, 4-1BB costimulatory domain, and intracellular CD3ζ signaling domain) and a RQR8 depletion ligand that makes the cells susceptible to rituximab. UCART123 exhibited both potent responses and persistence in a PDX model of primary BPDCN. These findings were highly encouraging for translating CD123CAR T cell immunotherapy into clinical settings.

The authors' group and others have examined or are currently examining CD123CAR T cell immunotherapy in clinical trials for both BPDCN and AML.[32,40] In the authors' ongoing phase 1 clinical trial at City of Hope (NCT02159495), the primary objectives are to test the safety and efficacy of CD123CAR T cells for patients with relapsed and/or refractory (r/r) AML (arm 1) and BPDCN (arm 2) and to determine the recommended phase 2 dose (RP2D). Autologous patient-derived CD123CAR T cells are infused as a salvage therapy, allowing the patients to achieve maximum regression before receiving an optional allo-HCT.[52] To date, 18 patients have been enrolled and 9 have been treated with CD123CAR T cell therapy on this trial. In the AML arm, all 7 patients had received 4 to 10 lines of prior treatment and at least one prior allo-HCT. (1) Two patients were treated at dose level 1 (50×10^6 CAR T cells) and 1 patient achieved morphologic leukemia-free state (MLFS). This patient received a second CAR T infusion and had a reduction of leukemic blasts from 77.9% to 0.9% using flow cytometric–based analysis. (2) Five patients were treated at dose level 2 (200×10^6 CAR T cells): 1 patient achieved CR with incomplete count recovery (CRi) and 1 patient achieved MLFS that improved to CR; the other 3 patients had stable disease. In the BPDCN arm, 2 patients were treated with 100×10^6 CAR T cells. One patient achieved CR with no evidence of CD123-, CD4-, or CD56-positive blasts in bone marrow or skin on day 28. The other patient remained in CR. Importantly, patients in both arms tolerated the treatment well and presented reversible toxicities, with no grade ≥ 3 cytokine release syndrome (CRS). Interim results of this trial were presented at the 2017 American Society of Hematology Annual Meeting[32] and the 2018 American Association of Cancer Research Special Conference on Tumor Immunology and Immunotherapy.[53] In December 2018, the FDA granted orphan drug designation to the City of Hope CD123CAR T cell product for the treatment of patients with AML and BPDCN. Taken together, the feasibility and safety of targeting CD123 using CAR T cell therapy has been demonstrated, with no myeloablative effects observed, for patients with r/r AML and BPDCN.

The University of Pennsylvania (Upenn) conducted a phase 1 trial using infusion of so-called biodegradable CART123 cells to treat patients with r/r AML (NCT02623582). In brief, to generate CART123 cells, autologous T cells were electroporated with CD123CAR mRNA, allowing the CART123 cells to express the CD123-targeting CAR for a limited period of time (ie, biodegradable). To test efficacy and short-term toxicities, patients in 2 cohorts received 3 to 6 infusions of 4×10^6 cell/kg CART123 cells. Nevertheless, CART123 cells exhibited limited antileukemic responses,[40] which resulted in termination of this phase 1 trial. In December 2018, Upenn initiated another phase 1 trial of second-generation CART123 cells that were generated using lentiviral delivery (NCT03766126). To address the severe concerns of myeloablation following CART123 cell therapy, as had been observed in preclinical studies,[49] patients on this trial may be treated with the T cell–depleting agent alemtuzumab[54] in the conditioning regimen before rescue allo-HCT subsequent to CART123 cell infusion. This phase 1 trial is ongoing and the results have yet to be published.

The MD Anderson Cancer Center and Cellectis performed two phase 1 clinical trials to test UCART123 cells[50,55] for the treatment of patients with r/r BPDCN (NCT03203369) and AML (NCT03190278). In the BPDCN trial, the first treated patient presented with skin lesions and 30% bone marrow blasts. Following infusion of 6.25×10^5 UCART123 cells/kg, the patient developed CRS and capillary leak syndrome (CLS) and died on day 9 post infusion. The BPDCN trial was subsequently closed for lack of sponsor support. In the AML trial, the first treated patient presented with 84% bone marrow blasts. Following infusion of 6.25×10^5 UCART123 cells/kg, the patient developed CRS and CLS, and was hospitalized in the intensive care unit.[56] The FDA allowed the AML trial to resume with an amended protocol that included 10-fold lower dosage of UCART123, reduced dose of the lymphodepletion regimen, and the establishment of an upper age limit of enrollment to 65 years old.[57,58] The AML trial is ongoing and the results have not yet been published.

RECOMBINANT FUSION PROTEIN: SL-401

SL-401 is a recombinant fusion protein consisting of human IL-3 (ligand of CD123) fused to truncated diphtheria toxin (DT) such that IL-3 replaces the domain of DT that binds to DT receptor. In this way, SL-401 can bind to CD123 via IL-3 and deliver DT to the cytosol of CD123[+] cells. When SL-401 binds to CD123 on BPDCN blasts the DT payload is internalized, where it inhibits protein synthesis and induces cell lysis. Encouraged by the 2013 trial by Frankel and colleagues[59] that demonstrated the safety and activity of SL-401 as a single agent for both BPDCN and AML, recent clinical studies have corroborated the durable responses and manageable toxicities of SL-401.[41,60,61] In December 2018, tagraxofusp (SL-401; Elzonris) received FDA approval for adults and children 2 years of age and older to treat BPDCN. SL-401 might also be a therapeutic option for patients with BPDCN who are not eligible for allo-HCT.[41,62] SL-401 is a proof of concept that targeting CD123 is feasible and efficacious for the treatment of BPDCN, and is reviewed in a separate article.

ANTIBODY-DRUG CONJUGATE: IMGN632

In addition to CD123CAR T cells and SL-401, other CD123-targeted immunotherapeutic approaches have been explored in both preclinical and clinical settings. IMGN632 is an ADC composed of a humanized monoclonal antibody (mAb) conjugated to a novel cytotoxic DNA-alkylating agent, indolinobenzodiazepine pseudodimer (IGN), via a peptide linker. IMGN632 binds to CD123[+] cells and is internalized along with IGN. Once inside the cell, IGN alkylates DNA without crosslinking and leads to CD123-specific lytic activity. In the preclinical setting, Zhang and colleagues[63] demonstrated that IMGN632 has potent antineoplastic activity against BPDCN in vitro and in vivo. Remarkably, IMGN632 shows activity even when given at a dosage that is 10-fold lower than the expected therapeutic dosage.

ImmunoGen is sponsoring an ongoing phase 1 clinical trial that aims to establish the maximum tolerated dose (MTD) and define the RP2D of IMGN632 for r/r patients with CD123[+] hematologic malignancies, including AML, BPDCN, and ALL (NCT03386513). Thus far, in the AML cohort 26% of the treated patients have achieved CR/CRi at a wide range of doses (0.015 mg/kg to 0.3 mg/kg). Importantly, no evidence of cumulative toxicity has been observed following up to 6 doses of IMGN632. Patients in the BPDCN cohort were treated with 0.045 mg/kg of IMGN632. Thus far, 2 out of 3 patients have shown a clinical response; 1 patient achieved partial response post treatment failure of SL-401 and 1 patient achieved unconfirmed CRi.[42] Taken together, IMGN632 demonstrates initial safety and activity for patients with r/r AML and BPDCN, and future studies are awaited for expansion cohorts and fractionated schedule.

BISPECIFIC ANTIBODY: XmAb14045

XmAb14045 is a BsAb composed of 2 antigen-binding domains: one that recognizes CD3 and one that recognizes CD123. XmAb14045 thus engages CD3-expressing endogenous T cells with CD123-expressing targets. Once engaged, T cells can be activated to mediate CD123-specific killing activity against target cells. In the preclinical setting, Chu and colleagues[64] demonstrated that XmAb14045 can effectively and safely deplete CD123$^+$ blasts in monkey peripheral blood and bone marrow at the doses of 1 and 10 µg/kg.

XmAb14045 is currently being evaluated in an ongoing phase 1 clinical trial sponsored by Xencor. The aims of the trial are to estimate the MTD or RP2D and schedule of XmAb14045 for the treatment of r/r patients with CD123$^+$ hematologic malignancies, including AML, BPDCN, B-ALL, and CML (NCT02730312). Ravandi and colleagues[43] presented initial results for patients with r/r AML treated with XmAb14045. Of the 64 patients treated, 77% experienced CRS (11% grade ≥3) and 23% achieved CR/CRi at the 1.3- and 2.3-µg/kg doses on the weekly dosing schedule. In February 2019, the FDA placed a partial hold on the trial because 2 patient deaths were considered at least possibly related to the treatment with XmAb14045.[65] One patient experienced severe CRS (grade ≥3[43]) following the first dose and another patient developed acute pulmonary edema (APE) following several doses of XmAb14045. Results for r/r patients with BPDCN, B-ALL, and CML have not yet been published. Taken together, XmAb14045 demonstrates clinical activity for patients with r/r AML, and CRS is the primary toxicity of XmAb14045 that needs careful management.

POTENTIAL RESISTANCE MECHANISM

Although the aforementioned immunotherapies have shown promising results for BPDCN treatment, several resistance mechanisms shed light on future combinational strategies to improve CD123-targeted therapies. Antigen loss is a common escape mechanism for any immunotherapy targeting a single antigen, including CD123-targeted immunotherapy. Cai and colleagues[50] found the appearance of CD123$^-$ BPDCN cells in all groups of UCART123-treated mice. This antigen loss resulted in escape from CD123-targeted therapy and early relapse.[50] Thus, there is a need to develop targeted therapies against other BPDCN-associated antigens. Currently a phase 2 clinical trial has opened for CD56$^+$ malignancies, including BPDCN, using lorvotuzumab mertansine (NCT02420873). Lorvotuzumab mertansine is an ADC that includes CD56 mAb conjugated to cytotoxic maytansine. Once bound to CD56$^+$ cells and the conjugate is subsequently internalized, maytansine inhibits tubulin polymerization that leads to cell death.[2,66,67] Therefore, future attention might be paid on dual-targeting to overcome antigen escape, including potentially targeting CD56 concurrently with CD123.

Another resistance mechanism was described by Stephansky and colleagues,[68] who demonstrated that SL-401 resistance is correlated with loss of *DPH1*, a diphthamide synthesis pathway enzyme, which can be silenced by DNA methylation. Specifically, SL-401 resistant clones showed significantly reduced expression of *DPH1*, and inverse correlation between SL-401 IC$_{50}$ (half-maximal inhibitory concentration) and *DPH1* levels was confirmed. In addition, CD45$^+$CD123$^+$ sorted AML blasts exhibited significantly decreased *DPH1* expression following SL-401 treatment. However, azacitidine, a hypomethylating agent approved for elderly patients with AML,[69] can reverse the DNA methylation and restore sensitivity to SL-401.[68] Therefore, a phase 1 clinical trial is ongoing to combine SL-401 and azacitidine for patients with AML or MDS (NCT03113643).

CHECKPOINT BLOCKADE: NIVOLUMAB

Checkpoint blockade targeting programmed death-1 (PD-1)/programmed death-ligand 1 (PD-L1) has remarkably changed the therapeutic landscape of solid tumors.[70–72] However, the clinical success of checkpoint blockade as a monotherapy to treat myeloid malignancies has been modest to date.[73,74] PD-L1 is expressed on malignant cells and antigen-presenting cells, where it can suppress T cell activation through interaction with PD-1 on T cells.[75] Aung and colleagues[76] have detected expression of PD-L1 on neoplastic cells using IHC in 10 of 21 patients (47.6%) with BPDCN, suggesting the therapeutic potential of checkpoint blockade targeting PD-1/PD-L1 interaction.

Nivolumab is an anti-PD-1 mAb that blocks PD-1 and prevents PD-1 on T cells from binding to PD-L1 on cancer cells. Thus, blocking this interaction might unleash the human immune system to destroy the cancer cells. Recently, nivolumab has received FDA approval for metastatic melanoma, renal cell carcinoma, non–small cell lung cancer, and classic Hodgkin lymphoma. Currently a phase 2 clinical trial is ongoing to characterize how patients with r/r peripheral T cell lymphoma and BPDCN respond to nivolumab (NCT03075553), with the results yet to be published.

SUMMARY

Recently, both clinical and research interests have focused on developing CD123-targeted immunotherapies for myeloid malignancies, particularly BPDCN and AML. CD123 is an attractive target given its aberrant expression on BPDCN and AML blasts compared with normal HSCs and myeloid progenitors. Encouraged by successful clinical translation of CD123CAR T cells and SL-401, other immunotherapies targeting CD123, including ADC and BsAb, are under active development for the treatment of BPDCN and other CD123+ hematologic malignancies. While we are waiting for the mature results from these studies, considerations need to be given to emergent observations that may affect the success of CD123-targeted immunotherapies. Future studies combining CD123CAR T cell therapy with other immunotherapies, such as checkpoint blockade, might lead to a superior antineoplastic response and improve the survival rate for patients with BPDCN and related CD123+ neoplasms.

DISCLOSURE

The authors have nothing to disclose.

CONFLICT OF INTEREST

The authors disclose no conflicts of interest.

REFERENCES

1. Sullivan JM, Rizzieri DA. Treatment of blastic plasmacytoid dendritic cell neoplasm. Hematologist 2016;16–23. https://doi.org/10.1182/asheducation-2016.1.16.
2. Falcone U, Sibai H, Deotare U. A critical review of treatment modalities for blastic plasmacytoid dendritic cell neoplasm. Crit Rev Oncol Hematol 2016;107:156–62.

3. Deotare U, Yee KW, Le LW, et al. Blastic plasmacytoid dendritic cell neoplasm with leukemic presentation: 10-Color flow cytometry diagnosis and HyperCVAD therapy. Am J Hematol 2016;91:283–6.

4. Vardiman JW, Thiele J, Arber DA, et al. The 2008 revision of the World Health Organization (WHO) classification of myeloid neoplasms and acute leukemia: rationale and important changes. Blood 2009;114:937–51.

5. Arber DA, Orazi A, Hasserjian R, et al. The 2016 revision to the World Health Organization classification of myeloid neoplasms and acute leukemia. Blood 2016; 127:2391–405.

6. Kharfan-Dabaja MA, Lazarus HM, Nishihori T, et al. Diagnostic and therapeutic advances in blastic plasmacytoid dendritic cell neoplasm: a focus on hematopoietic cell transplantation. Biol Blood Marrow Transplant 2013;19:1006–12.

7. Herling M, Jones D. CD41/CD561 hematodermic tumor: the features of an evolving entity and its relationship to dendritic cells. Am J Clin Pathol 2007; 127:687–700.

8. Jacob MC, Chaperot L, Mossuz P, et al. CD4+ CD56+ lineage negative malignancies: a new entity developed from malignant early plasmacytoid dendritic cells. Haematologica 2003;88:941–55.

9. Bekkenk MW, Jansen PM, Meijer CJ, et al. CD561 hematological neoplasms presenting in the skin: a retrospective analysis of 23 new cases and 130 cases from the literature. Ann Oncol 2004;15:1097–108.

10. Lucioni M, Novara F, Fiandrino G, et al. Twenty-one cases of blastic plasmacytoid dendritic cell neoplasm: focus on biallelic locus 9p21.3 deletion. Blood 2011;118: 4591–4.

11. Laribi K, Denizon N, Besancon A, et al. Blastic plasmacytoid dendritic cell neoplasm: from origin of the cell to targeted therapies. Biol Blood Marrow Transplant 2016;22:1357–67.

12. Betrian S, Guenounou S, Luquet I, et al. Bendamustine for relapsed blastic plasmacytoid dendritic cell leukaemia. Hematol Oncol 2017;35:252–5.

13. Xie W, Zhao Y, Cao L, et al. Cutaneous blastic plasmacytoid dendritic cell neoplasm occurring after spontaneous remission of acute myeloid leukemia: a case report and review of literature. Med Oncol 2012;29:2417–22.

14. Martin-Martin L, Lopez A, Vidriales B, et al. Classification and clinical behavior of blastic plasmacytoid dendritic cell neoplasms according to their maturation-associated immunophenotypic profile. Oncotarget 2015;6:19204–16.

15. Feuillard J, Jacob MC, Valensi F, et al. Clinical and biologic features of CD4(+) CD56(+) malignancies. Blood 2002;99:1556–63.

16. Julia F, Petrella T, Beylot-Barry M, et al. Blastic plasmacytoid dendritic cell neoplasm: clinical features in 90 patients. Br J Dermatol 2013;169:579–86.

17. Cota C, Vale E, Viana I, et al. Cutaneous manifestations of blastic plasmacytoid dendritic cell neoplasm-morphologic and phenotypic variability in a series of 33 patients. Am J Surg Pathol 2010;34:75–87.

18. Khoury JD, Medeiros LJ, Manning JT, et al. CD56(+) TdT(+) blastic natural killer cell tumor of the skin: a primitive systemic malignancy related to myelomonocytic leukemia. Cancer 2002;94:2401–8.

19. Herling M, Teitell MA, Shen RR, et al. TCL1 expression in plasmacytoid dendritic cells (DC2s) and the related CD41 CD561 blastic tumors of skin. Blood 2003;101: 5007–9.

20. Kazakov DV, Mentzel T, Burg G, et al. Blastic natural killer-cell lymphoma of the skin associated with myelodysplastic syndrome or myelogenous leukaemia: a coincidence or more? Br J Dermatol 2003;149:869–76.

21. Brunetti L, Di Battista V, Venanzi A, et al. Blastic plasmacytoid dendritic cell neoplasm and chronic myelomonocytic leukemia: a shared clonal origin. Leukemia 2017;31:1238–40.
22. Sangle NA, Schmidt RL, Patel JL, et al. Optimized immunohistochemical panel to differentiate myeloid sarcoma from blastic plasmacytoid dendritic cell neoplasm. Mod Pathol 2014;27:1137–43.
23. Roos-Weil D, Dietrich S, Boumendil A, et al. Stem cell transplantation can provide durable disease control in blastic plasmacytoid dendritic cell neoplasm: a retrospective study from the European Group for Blood and Marrow Transplantation. Blood 2013;121:440–6.
24. Pagano L, Valentini CG, Grammatico S, et al. Blastic plasmacytoid dendritic cell neoplasm: diagnostic criteria and therapeutical approaches. Br J Haematol 2016; 174:188–202.
25. Kim MJ, Nasr A, Kabir B, et al. Pediatric blastic plasmacytoid dendritic cell neoplasm: a systematic literature review. J Pediatr Hematol Oncol 2017;39: 528–37.
26. Kerr D 2nd, Sokol L. The advances in therapy of blastic plasmacytoid dendritic cell neoplasm. Expert Opin Investig Drugs 2018;27:733–9.
27. Pagano L, Valentini CG, Pulsoni A, et al. Blastic plasmacytoid dendritic cell neoplasm with leukemic presentation: an Italian multicenter study. Haematologica 2013;98:239–46.
28. Testa U, Pelosi E, Frankel A. CD 123 is a membrane biomarker and a therapeutic target in hematologic malignancies. Biomark Res 2014;2:4.
29. Ehninger A, Kramer M, Rollig C, et al. Distribution and levels of cell surface expression of CD33 and CD123 in acute myeloid leukemia. Blood Cancer J 2014;4:e218.
30. Garnache-Ottou F, Feuillard J, Ferrand C, et al. Extended diagnostic criteria for plasmacytoid dendritic cell leukaemia. Br J Haematol 2009;145:624–36.
31. Jordan CT, Upchurch D, Szilvassy SJ, et al. The interleukin-3 receptor alpha chain is a unique marker for human acute myelogenous leukemia stem cells. Leukemia 2000;14:1777–84.
32. Budde L, Song JY, Kim Y, et al. Remissions of acute myeloid leukemia and blastic plasmacytoid dendritic cell neoplasm following treatment with CD123-specific CAR T cells: a first-in-human clinical trial. Blood 2017;130:811.
33. Testa U, Riccioni R, Militi S, et al. Elevated expression of IL-3Ralpha in acute myelogenous leukemia is associated with enhanced blast proliferation, increased cellularity, and poor prognosis. Blood 2002;100:2980–8.
34. Chaperot L, Bendriss N, Manches O, et al. Identification of a leukemic counterpart of the plasmacytoid dendritic cells. Blood 2001;97:3210–7.
35. Munoz L, Nomdedeu JF, Lopez O, et al. Interleukin-3 receptor alpha chain (CD123) is widely expressed in hematologic malignancies. Haematologica 2001;86:1261–9.
36. Aldinucci D, Olivo K, Lorenzon D, et al. The role of interleukin-3 in classical Hodgkin's disease. Leuk Lymphoma 2005;46:303–11.
37. Frolova O, Benito J, Brooks C, et al. SL-401 and SL-501, targeted therapeutics directed at the interleukin-3 receptor, inhibit the growth of leukaemic cells and stem cells in advanced phase chronic myeloid leukaemia. Br J Haematol 2014; 166:862–74.
38. Du X, Ho M, Pastan I. New immunotoxins targeting CD123, a stem cell antigen on acute myeloid leukemia cells. J Immunother 2007;30:607–13.

39. Jin L, Lee EM, Ramshaw HS, et al. Monoclonal antibody-mediated targeting of CD123, IL-3 receptor alpha chain, eliminates human acute myeloid leukemic stem cells. Cell Stem Cell 2009;5:31–42.

40. Cummins KD, Frey N, Nelson AM, et al. Treating relapsed/refractory (RR) AML with biodegradable anti-CD123 CAR modified T cells. Blood 2017;130:1359.

41. Pemmaraju N, Lane AA, Sweet KL, et al. Tagraxofusp in blastic plasmacytoid dendritic-cell neoplasm. N Engl J Med 2019;380:1628–37.

42. Daver NG, Erba HP, Papadantonakis N, et al. A phase I, first-in-human study evaluating the safety and preliminary antileukemia activity of IMGN632, a novel CD123-targeting antibody-drug conjugate, in patients with relapsed/refractory acute myeloid leukemia and other CD123-positive hematologic malignancies. Blood 2018;132:27.

43. Ravandi F, Bashey A, Foran JM, et al. Complete responses in relapsed/refractory acute myeloid leukemia (AML) patients on a weekly dosing schedule of XmAb14045, a CD123 × CD3 T cell-engaging bispecific antibody: initial results of a phase 1 study. Blood 2018;132:763.

44. Kalos M, Levine BL, Porter DL, et al. T cells with chimeric antigen receptors have potent antitumor effects and can establish memory in patients with advanced leukemia. Sci Transl Med 2011;3:95ra73.

45. Scholler J, Brady TL, Binder-Scholl G, et al. Decade-long safety and function of retroviral-modified chimeric antigen receptor T cells. Sci Transl Med 2012;4:132ra153.

46. Schuster SJ, Svoboda J, Chong EA, et al. Chimeric antigen receptor T cells in refractory B-cell lymphomas. N Engl J Med 2017;377:2545–54.

47. Schuster SJ, Bishop MR, Tam CS, et al. Tisagenlecleucel in adult relapsed or refractory diffuse large B-cell lymphoma. N Engl J Med 2019;380:45–56.

48. Mardiros A, Dos Santos C, McDonald T, et al. T cells expressing CD123-specific chimeric antigen receptors exhibit specific cytolytic effector functions and antitumor effects against human acute myeloid leukemia. Blood 2013;122:3138–48.

49. Gill S, Tasian SK, Ruella M, et al. Preclinical targeting of human acute myeloid leukemia and myeloablation using chimeric antigen receptor-modified T cells. Blood 2014;123:2343–54.

50. Cai T, Galetto R, Gouble A, et al. Pre-clinical studies of anti-CD123 CAR-T cells for the treatment of blastic plasmacytoid dendritic cell neoplasm (BPDCN). Blood 2016;128:4039.

51. Wang X, Chang WC, Wong CW, et al. A transgene-encoded cell surface polypeptide for selection, in vivo tracking, and ablation of engineered cells. Blood 2011;118:1255–63.

52. Mardiros A, Forman SJ, Budde LE. T cells expressing CD123 chimeric antigen receptors for treatment of acute myeloid leukemia. Curr Opin Hematol 2015;22:484–8.

53. Budde L. CD123CAR displays clincal activity in relapsed/refractory (r/r) acute myeloid leukemia (AML) and blastic plasmacytoid dendritic cell neoplasm (BPDCN): safety and efficacy results from a phase 1 study. Poster Session B22, Tumor Immunology and Immunotherapy, AACR (2018). Miami Beach, November 30, 2018.

54. Tasian SK, Kenderian SS, Shen F, et al. Optimized depletion of chimeric antigen receptor T cells in murine xenograft models of human acute myeloid leukemia. Blood 2017;129:2395–407.

55. Cai T, Black KL, Naqvi A, et al. Preclinical efficacy of allogeneic anti-CD123 CAR T-cells for the therapy of blastic plasmacytoid dendritic cell neoplasm (BPDCN). Cancer Res 2018;78:2560.

56. Cellectis. 2017. Available at: http://www.cellectis.com/en/press/fda-lifts-clinicalhold-on-cellectis-phase-1-clinical-trials-with-ucart123-in-aml-and-bpdcn. Accessed September 24, 2019.

57. Testa U, Pelosi E, Castelli G. CD123 as a therapeutic target in the treatment of hematological malignancies. Cancers (Basel) 2019;11. https://doi.org/10.3390/cancers11091358.

58. Cummins KD, Gill S. Chimeric antigen receptor T-cell therapy for acute myeloid leukemia: how close to reality? Haematologica 2019;104:1302.

59. Frankel AE, Konopleva M, Hogge D, et al. Activity and tolerability of SL-401, a targeted therapy directed to the interleukin-3 receptor on cancer stem cells and tumor bulk, as a single agent in patients with advanced hematologic malignancies. J Clin Oncol 2013;31:7029.

60. Pemmaraju N, Sweet KL, Lane AA, et al. Results of pivotal phase 2 trial of SL-401 in patients with blastic plasmacytoid dendritic cell neoplasm (BPDCN). Blood 2017;130:1298.

61. Frankel AE, Woo JH, Ahn C, et al. Activity of SL-401, a targeted therapy directed to interleukin-3 receptor, in blastic plasmacytoid dendritic cell neoplasm patients. Blood 2014;124:385–92.

62. Kerr D 2nd, Zhang L, Sokol L. Blastic plasmacytoid dendritic cell neoplasm. Curr Treat Options Oncol 2019;20:9.

63. Zhang Q, Cai T, Han L, et al. Pre-clinical efficacy of CD123-targeting antibody-drug conjugate IMGN632 in blastic plasmacytoid dendritic cell neoplasm (BPDCN) models. Blood 2018;132:3956.

64. Chu SY, Pong E, Chen H, et al. Immunotherapy with long-lived anti-CD123 × anti-CD3 bispecific antibodies stimulates potent T cell-mediated killing of human AML cell lines and of CD123+ cells in monkeys: a potential therapy for acute myelogenous leukemia. Blood 2014;124:2316.

65. Xencor. 2019. Available at: https://investors.xencor.com/news-releases/newsrelease-details/xencor-announces-partial-clinical-hold-phase-1-study-xmab14045. Accessed September 24, 2019.

66. Tassone P, Gozzini A, Goldmacher V, et al. In vitro and in vivo activity of the maytansinoid immunoconjugate huN901-N2′-deacetyl-N2′-(3-mercapto-1-oxopropyl)-maytansine against CD56+ multiple myeloma cells. Cancer Res 2004; 64:4629–36.

67. Remillard S, Rebhun LI, Howie GA, et al. Antimitotic activity of the potent tumor inhibitor maytansine. Science 1975;189:1002–5.

68. Togami K, Pastika T, Stephansky J. DNA methyltransferase inhibition overcomes diphthamide pathway deficiencies underlying CD123-targeted treatment resistance. J Clin Invest 2019;129(11):5005–19.

69. DiNardo CD, Pratz K, Pullarkat V, et al. Venetoclax combined with decitabine or azacitidine in treatment-naive, elderly patients with acute myeloid leukemia. Blood 2019;133:7–17.

70. Couzin-Frankel J. Breakthrough of the year 2013. Cancer immunotherapy. Science 2013;342:1432–3.

71. Dizon DS, Krilov L, Cohen E, et al. Clinical cancer advances 2016: annual report on progress against cancer from the American Society of Clinical Oncology. J Clin Oncol 2016;34:987–1011.

72. Pardoll DM. The blockade of immune checkpoints in cancer immunotherapy. Nat Rev Cancer 2012;12:252–64.
73. Berger R, Rotem-Yehudar R, Slama G, et al. Phase I safety and pharmacokinetic study of CT-011, a humanized antibody interacting with PD-1, in patients with advanced hematologic malignancies. Clin Cancer Res 2008;14:3044–51.
74. Boddu P, Kantarjian H, Garcia-Manero G, et al. The emerging role of immune checkpoint based approaches in AML and MDS. Leuk Lymphoma 2018;59: 790–802.
75. Sun C, Mezzadra R, Schumacher TN. Regulation and function of the PD-L1 checkpoint. Immunity 2018;48:434–52.
76. Aung PP, Sukswai N, Nejati R, et al. PD1/PD-L1 expression in blastic plasmacytoid dendritic cell neoplasm. Cancers (Basel) 2019;11. https://doi.org/10.3390/cancers11050695.

Novel Therapies for Blastic Plasmacytoid Dendritic Cell Neoplasm

Andrew A. Lane, MD, PhD

KEYWORDS

- BPDCN • Tagraxofusp • Venetoclax • Azacitidine • BCL2 • Bromodomain • IDH
- FLT3

KEY POINTS

- Blastic plasmacytoid dendritic cell neoplasm (BPDCN) depends on BCL2 and is sensitive to BCL2 inhibition using venetoclax.
- Tagraxofusp (SL-401) resistance is caused by downregulation of the diphthamide synthesis pathway and loss of the target of diphtheria toxin; loss of CD123 is not common.
- Tagraxofusp resistance is reversible by azacitidine, and the combination of tagraxofusp with azacitidine is active in BPDCN models in vivo.
- Bromodomain and extraterminal domain inhibitors and liver X receptor agonists are active in preclinical studies of BPDCN.
- IDH1, IDH2, FLT3, and RNA splicing factor mutations are present in BPDCN and may indicate therapeutic opportunities using drugs that have been tested in other malignancies.

INTRODUCTION

Blastic plasmacytoid dendritic cell neoplasm (BPDCN) is an orphan, aggressive hematologic malignancy of unmet clinical need.[1-3] Outcomes are poor, with median overall survival of 2 years or less.[4,5] The first targeted therapy for BPDCN, tagraxofusp, a recombinant fusion protein of interleukin 3 (IL3) to a truncated diphtheria toxin, was approved by the United States Food and Drug Administration in December 2018.[6-8] Approval was based on a high complete and overall response rate in a phase 2 trial,[9] and tagraxofusp is widely becoming a standard first-line treatment of BPDCN in the United States. Despite this success, there remains an ongoing need to identify additional agents with activity in BPDCN. As of this writing, tagraxofusp was approved only in the United States, highlighting the need for other active drugs with wider availability. Also, a minority of the BPDCN population is not eligible for tagraxofusp due to comorbidities or does not respond to the drug. There are also patients who relapse after

BPDCN Center, Dana-Farber Cancer Institute, Harvard Medical School, 450 Brookline Avenue, Mayer 413, Boston, MA 02215, USA
E-mail address: andrew_lane@dfci.harvard.edu
Twitter: @lane_andy (A.A.L.)

Hematol Oncol Clin N Am 34 (2020) 589–600
https://doi.org/10.1016/j.hoc.2020.01.007
0889-8588/20/© 2020 Elsevier Inc. All rights reserved.

having an initial response to tagraxofusp or relapse after stem cell transplantation. For all of these reasons, investigators are actively exploring therapeutic vulnerabilities in BPDCN that might offer additional options for patients.

The target for tagraxofusp is the IL3 receptor, which is composed of a unique alpha chain (IL3-Rα), also called CD123, and a common beta chain (βc, **Fig. 1**). CD123 is highly expressed on the cell surface of all BPDCNs and therefore is an attractive target.[10] Other articles in this issue will discuss the research that led to tagraxofusp approval and other agents targeting CD123 that are in development. These include antibody-drug conjugates, bispecific CD3 x CD123 T-cell engagers, and CAR-T cells.[11,12] Other molecules expressed on the surface of BPDCN cells, such as CD56 and LILRB4/ILT3, are targets of immunotherapies being tested in other diseases that might also be applied to BPDCN (see **Fig. 1**).[13–15]

In this review, the author focuses on small molecule therapeutics with potential in BPDCN. They also discuss recent data regarding the mechanism of resistance to tagraxofusp and combination strategies being used to overcome resistance and enhance tagraxofusp efficacy.

BPDCN GENETICS HAVE NOT YET REVEALED A UNIVERSALLY SHARED THERAPEUTIC TARGET

There is no defining molecular lesion found in all cases of BPDCN discovered to date. DNA copy number analyses revealed recurrent loss of cell-cycle regulators, such as

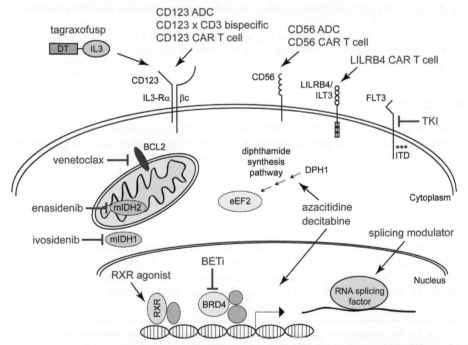

Fig. 1. Novel targets and agents in BPDCN. Emerging strategies for treating BPDCN discussed in this article are shown. ADC, antibody-drug conjugate; BETi, bromodomain and extraterminal motif inhibitor; CAR, chimeric antigen receptor; DT, diphtheria toxin; eEF2, eukaryotic elongation factor 2; IL3, interleukin 3; mIDH1 and mIDH2, mutant isocitrate dehydrogenase 1 and 2; RXR, retinoid X receptor; TKI, tyrosine kinase inhibitor. ***ITD, internal tandem duplication mutation in FLT3.

CDKN2A and RB1.[16–18] Additional studies have reported other targets of structural alteration, such as ETV6,[19,20]MYC,[21,22] and the transcription factor MYB that interestingly is weighted toward pediatric patients.[23] However, none of these abnormalities are immediately therapeutically targetable and do not implicate a universal vulnerability in BPDCN cells.

DNA sequencing studies have been reported in a relatively small number of BPDCN cases. The pattern of mutated genes is highly overlapping with other myeloid malignancies, such as myelodysplastic syndrome (MDS), chronic myelomonocytic leukemia, and acute myeloid leukemia (AML).[24–26] These genes include TET2, ASXL1, TP53, NRAS, KRAS, and those that encode RNA splicing factors. None are uniformly mutated across all BPDCNs, nor are there approved drugs to target these mutations, with the exception of a few examples that are discussed later.

BPDCN DEPENDS ON BCL2 AND IS SENSITIVE TO THE BCL2 INHIBITOR VENETOCLAX

Given there are not (yet) any DNA mutations that are universally targetable in most BPDCNs, the author pursued other dependencies. The BCL2 gene, encoding an antiapoptotic cell survival protein, is overexpressed in BPDCN.[27,28] However, expression of BCL2 does not necessarily equate with dependency on the BCL2 protein.[29] Thus, functional analyses of mitochondrial apoptosis were employed to determine which survival pathways were most active in BPDCN cells.[28] Specifically, they used BH3 profiling, an ex vivo measurement of cytochrome c release or mitochondrial outer membrane permeabilization in tumor cells stimulated with synthetic BH3 domain–containing peptides.[30] These peptides are activators of mitochondrial apoptosis and indicate the propensity of a cell to die after stimulation of specific apoptosis pathway components. BH3 profiling is also amenable to flow cytometry–based assessment, which facilitates single-cell resolution of BPDCN cells separated from surrounding normal tissue.[31]

These experiments found that BPDCNs highly depend on BCL2 for survival.[28] This dependency was present across numerous primary BPDCNs and patient-derived xenografts (PDXs), and in all cases they exhibited greater BCL2 dependency than AMLs or normal healthy donor bone marrow controls. Furthermore, unlike many other cell types, BPDCNs almost solely depended on BCL2, suggesting that if BCL2 was inhibited the cells would not be able to rely on alternative antiapoptotic proteins for survival. As predicted by these results, BPDCNs were highly sensitive to BCL2 inhibition using the small molecule inhibitor venetoclax. The in vitro GI50 (concentration at which growth is 50% of control) for venetoclax in BPDCN of ~10 nM is similar with that in chronic lymphocytic leukemia (CLL), a disease where the drug has high single-agent activity.[32] The reason for this striking BCL2 dependence is not obvious. There are no DNA mutations or rearrangements involving BCL2 reported in BPDCN. It is possible that BCL2 dependency is related to the pDC lineage relationship of BPDCN, given that survival of mouse pDCs, but not conventional DCs, in vivo also depended on BCL2.[33]

To test for in vivo therapeutic relevance of these observations, animals bearing BPDCN PDXs were treated with venetoclax, which resulted in a significant decrease in leukemia burden in blood, bone marrow, and spleen and prolonged overall survival compared with controls. Then, in a pilot study, the author treated 2 patients with relapsed BPDCN using single-agent venetoclax. Both had significant clinical responses, despite having failed 4 to 5 prior lines of therapy including stem cell transplantation. Although these responses were relatively short-lived (less than 3 months), these results suggested that venetoclax has clinically relevant activity in

BPDCN. Since that time, several other reports of response to venetoclax in BPDCN have been published, using the drug alone or in combination.[34–37] The author has initiated a formal phase 1 clinical trial of venetoclax in BPDCN (ClinicalTrials.gov: NCT03485547), which will establish dosing and safety parameters and will facilitate future combination trials with tagraxofusp or other agents.

COMBINATIONS WITH TAGRAXOFUSP

Another strategy for development of novel agents in BPDCN is to combine drugs with tagraxofusp. Although highly effective, tagraxofusp fails in a subset of BPDCNs, and even among those who achieve remission, some patients relapse after stem cell transplantation. One tactic is to identify other agents with activity in the disease, such as venetoclax, and empirically test combinations. These are currently being pursued in the laboratory and in clinical trials, as outlined later. As an alternative approach, in a recent project the author attempted to improve tagraxofusp efficacy by asking what determines resistance to the drug and how might it be overcome therapeutically.[38]

The initial hypothesis was that there would be decreased expression or alteration of the target (CD123) in the setting of resistance, as has been reported for CD19- and CD22-targeted therapies in B-cell malignancies.[39,40] However, they did not observe any instances of CD123 loss on the surface of patients' BPDCN cells during or after treatment with tagraxofusp. This was also true in laboratory models, including BPDCN and AML cell lines and PDXs. Loss-of-function assays have suggested that myeloid leukemia cells have a growth disadvantage after CD123 depletion,[41] which may, in part, drive them to alternative resistance pathways.

Instead of CD123 loss causing tagraxofusp resistance, BPDCN and AML cells became insensitive to the cytotoxic effects of diphtheria toxin. This was mediated by downregulation of components of the diphthamide synthesis pathway, particularly *DPH1*, which is responsible for conversion of histidine 715 on eukaryotic elongation factor 2 (eEF2) to a variant amino acid called diphthamide.[42] Diphthamide 715 is the target for ADP-ribosylation by diphtheria toxin, which, when modified, results in eEF2 inhibition, blockade of protein synthesis, and cell death. In other words, tagraxofusp resistance was associated with loss of the intracellular target of diphtheria toxin.

DPH1 downregulation was associated with hypermethylation of DNA CpG islands in the *DPH1* gene promoter region, a DNA modification associated with gene silencing. When treated with noncytotoxic doses of the DNA methyltransferase inhibitor 5-azacitidine (azacitidine), resistant cells showed reduced *DPH1* locus DNA methylation, increased *DPH1* expression, and resensitization to tagraxofusp. In parallel, BH3 profiling was used to determine if tagraxofusp-resistant cells had lost the ability to undergo apoptosis. Unlike the decreased apoptotic priming that is characteristic of resistance to many cancer drugs,[43,44] they found that tagraxofusp resistance was instead associated with increased apoptotic priming and increased sensitivity to cytotoxic chemotherapy. This included drugs active in BPDCN, such as anthracyclines, cytarabine, and vincristine, as well as cytotoxic doses of azacitidine. Naïve BPDCN and AML cells also demonstrated synergistic, rather than simply additive, cell killing with combinations of tagraxofusp and chemotherapy.[38]

Together, these data support clinical testing of tagraxofusp together with conventional cytotoxic agents. They also suggest that the specific combination of tagraxofusp and azacitidine might be particularly active in BPDCN. Based on these findings, the author predicted that up-front combination of the 2 drugs would cause synergistic cell death, and, azacitidine's effects on DNA methylation could restore tagraxofusp sensitivity to cells that escape via diphthamide pathway downregulation.

Consistent with this hypothesis, in vivo treatment of BPDCN PDXs was more effective with the combination of tagraxofusp and azacitidine over either agent alone and resulted in measurable residual disease (MRD) negativity in most of the animals.[38]

Other studies have also provided evidence that DNA methyltransferase inhibitors are active in BPDCN. Two case series reported a total of 5 patients treated with azacitidine and all had some clinical benefit.[45,46] In the laboratory, Sapienza and colleagues[24] determined that BPDCNs may be driven by deranged gene expression control, as evidenced by mutations in epigenome regulators and altered patterns of chromatin modification linked to specific cancer genes. They also tested several epigenome-modifying drugs in a cell line model of BPDCN in vivo and found that the DNA methyltransferase inhibitors azacitidine and decitabine were particularly active.

Considering all of these data, the author initiated a multicenter phase 1 trial of the combination of tagraxofusp and azacitidine, given in an overlapping schedule (ClinicalTrials.gov: NCT03113643). The objectives of the trial are to determine the safe dose and schedule the combination and to obtain a preliminary estimate of efficacy. Accompanying correlative studies in the laboratory will measure associations with response including gene expression and diphthamide synthesis pathway activity. The trial is open for patients with high-risk myeloid malignancies (AML or MDS with >10% bone marrow blasts) and is planned to expand to patients with BPDCN in the near future.

TRANSCRIPTION FACTORS AND EPIGENETIC MACHINERY AS TARGETS

Another strategy to target BPDCN is to exploit transcriptional dependencies that are inherent in dendritic cells or acquired during transformation. Ceribelli and colleagues[41] performed an RNA interference screen in a BPDCN cell line and identified the transcription factor TCF4 as the top hit that decreased viability when knocked down. Similar to BCL2, it is possible that this represents a lineage-defined dependency, as TCF4 (also known as E2-2) is known to be required for dendritic cell development and function.[47,48] Accordingly, TCF4 knockdown abrogated pDC and BPDCN-specific gene signatures, including downregulation of BCL2 and MYC, genes that are upregulated in BPDCNs compared with normal hematopoietic cells.[27,28]

Next, the investigators performed a drug screen that identified 3 bromodomain and extra-terminal (BET) domain inhibitors among the hits that were highly toxic to 2 BPDCN cell lines.[41] Of note, the BET family member BRD4, a direct target of BET inhibitors,[49] was also one of the top hits from the shRNA screen as a BPDCN-selective dependency. Treatment with BET inhibitors caused downregulation of TCF4 and disruption of a TCF4-associated "super-enhancer" landscape that was highly enriched for BPDCN-associated genes. Together, these data nominated TCF4 as a critical lineage-survival oncogene in BPDCN that might be targeted by BET inhibition.

Emadali and colleagues[50] took a different approach that also led to nomination of BET inhibitors as having therapeutic potential in BPDCN. They identified abnormalities of chromosome 5q in approximately one-third of BPDCNs. By mapping the commonly deleted region on 5q and a t(3;5)(q21;q31) translocation in one case, they focused on NR3C1, which encodes the glucocorticoid receptor GCR. Patients with BPDCN with 5q/NR3C1 deletion had poorer survival. NR3C1 deletion was associated with glucocorticoid resistance and upregulation of several leukemia-associated genes. They also characterized a long intergenic noncoding RNA (lincRNA) on 3q21 involved in the t(3;5), linc-RNA-3q. Linc-RNA-3q was upregulated in BPDCNs relative to normal pDCs (including in those without the translocation), and its expression correlated with cancer-associated transcriptional alterations. Treatment with the BET inhibitor JQ1 displaced BRD4 from the *linc-RNA-3q* promoter, decreased *linc-RNA-3q* expression, and impaired growth of a BPDCN cell line in a xenotransplantation assay in vivo.

Together, these 2 studies suggest that BET inhibitors disrupt critical transcriptional pathways in BPDCN cells, resulting in impaired growth or survival. Because several BET inhibitors are in clinical development as single agents or in combinations, including in other hematologic malignancies, these might be strategies to pursue in BPDCN. It is not yet clear if there is a biomarker for which specific BPDCNs would be most sensitive to BET inhibitors or if they would be broadly active.

A 2016 study of BPDCN transcriptomes identified the liver X receptor (LXR) pathway as a potentially important mediator of disease biology.[51] Downregulation of cholesterol homeostasis pathway genes, many of which are normally controlled by LXR, was a consistent feature unique to BPDCN, different from AML, T-cell acute lymphoblastic leukemia, and normal pDCs. LXR is a nuclear receptor for endogenous oxysterols and cholesterol biosynthesis intermediates.[52] Treatment of BPDCN cells with LXR agonists increased expression of LXR target genes and upregulated cholesterol efflux via membrane transporters. This was associated with G1 cell-cycle arrest and induction of apoptosis, with impaired survival signaling via STAT5 and nuclear factor kB (NF-kB) pathways. Treatment of mice bearing BPDCN cell line xenografts with an LXR agonist resulted in improved survival. LXR agonists are in trials in several diseases and could thus represent another transcriptionally directed therapy for application to BPDCN.

Recurrent chromosomal rearrangements in a subset of BPDCNs involve *MYC* and *MYB*, both of which encode protooncogene transcription factors that are activated in diverse cancers. *MYC*-rearranged BPDCNs occur in older patients and are associated with a poorer prognosis.[22,53] Although there are no direct MYC inhibitors in clinical use, BET inhibitors downregulate *MYC* expression and one study suggested that *MYC*-rearranged BPDCN cells were sensitive to BET inhibition.[22] *MYB* rearrangement was also observed in BPDCN, possibly more frequently in children.[23] Novel strategies to disrupt MYB function are in preclinical development[54] and thus might be applied to BPDCN, particularly for pediatric patients or those with *MYB* locus rearrangements.

DRUGS IN CLINICAL USE OR IN DEVELOPMENT FOR OTHER CANCERS

We may be able to adopt treatments for BPDCN that have been studied in other malignancies, using empirical or biomarker-driven patient selection. Bortezomib is a small-molecule proteasome inhibitor that is used in several blood cancers. Although bortezomib likely acts via multiple mechanisms, one that has received significant attention is its effect on the NF-kB pathway. BPDCNs have signatures of constitutive NF-kB activation and BPDCN cells are sensitive to an NF-kB p65 inhibitor.[27,51] Philippe and colleagues[55] showed that bortezomib treatment of BPDCN cells induced cell-cycle arrest, decreased viability when given alone, and enhanced cytotoxicity when combined with an anthracycline or azacitidine. Bortezomib was also active in vivo against a BPDCN PDX model, prolonging survival in association with impaired tumor cell NF-kB signaling.

These data raise the possibility that bortezomib may be active in BPDCN and support clinical evaluation. A recent case report described prolonged remission in a patient with BPDCN who received bortezomib and simvastatin followed by venetoclax.[36] Other bortezomib combinations may also be active in BPDCN. The thalidomide derivative lenalidomide induced apoptosis and reduced tumor burden in a PDX model of BPDCN.[56] Subsequent case series reported clinical remissions in patients following treatment with bortezomib and lenalidomide, with or without dexamethasone.[57,58]

Retrospective analyses have also pointed to other "conventional" cytotoxic chemotherapies that may have favorable activity in BPDCN. For example, several studies reported improved outcomes when "ALL-like" rather than "AML-like" or "lymphoma-like" chemotherapy regimens were used.[4,59] Whether specific drugs within these cocktails mediate differences in outcome is unknown. In an analysis of patients with BPDCN treated in the pre-tagraxofusp era at 3 US cancer centers, the author made a similar observation of better outcomes with lymphoid-type chemotherapy and also uncovered a cohort of 8 patients treated with the antifolate pralatrexate; 4 had complete responses, including in the relapsed disease setting.[4] Whether these differences in outcomes by chemotherapy type are due to treatment intensity, patient selection bias, or instead, intrinsic molecular properties of BPDCN is unclear. Identifying biomarkers of activity may be a fruitful area of study, as we should not discount the effect of conventional chemotherapy, even in this era of targeted treatment development.

Finally, although there is no BPDCN-specific genetic alteration that has been identified nor any genes that are consistently mutated across all cases, the spectrum of somatic mutations overlaps with other malignancies, particularly myeloid cancers. Therefore, DNA sequencing may offer another source for co-opting existing therapies for patients with BPDCN. For example, the metabolic enzymes isocitrate dehydrogenase (IDH) 1 and 2 are mutated in AML and other cancers and are the subject of intense preclinical and clinical research. This has resulted in 2 recent drug approvals of small-molecule IDH inhibitors for patients with AML harboring IDH1[60] or IDH2[61] mutations. IDH2 was mutated in 9% of BPDCNs in one series of 33 patients[26], and IDH1 in 4% and IDH2 in 12% in another series of 25 patients.[25] The author reported a patient with BPDCN harboring an IDH2 R140Q mutation who achieved a prolonged disease response during treatment with single-agent enasidenib, an approved IDH2 inhibitor.[4] Decreased variant allele frequency of the IDH2 mutation coincident with decreased BPDCN involvement in the bone marrow during treatment suggested on-target activity.

FMS-like tyrosine kinase 3 (FLT3) is a receptor tyrosine kinase that is activated by point mutation or internal tandem duplication (ITD) in a significant fraction of AMLs. Several FLT3 tyrosine kinase inhibitors (TKIs) are approved for AML and others are in development.[62] One study reported that 3 of 13 BPDCNs with normal karyotype harbored a FLT3-ITD mutation.[5] The author is not aware of any reports of patients with BPDCN receiving FLT3 TKIs, but these data suggest it may be a targetable molecular lesion as in AML. Lastly, RNA splicing genes such as SF3B1, SRSF2, U2AF1, and ZRSR2 are recurrently mutated in MDS, AML, and other hematologic malignancies, as well as in several types of solid tumors. Splicing modulator drugs may preferentially decrease viability of malignant cells that harbor these mutations[63] and several are in clinical development. BPDCN harbors the same splicing gene mutations, in 36% of cases in one report.[25] Thus, BPDCN may be relatively enriched for biomarker-positive cases and could represent another candidate malignancy for testing splicing modulator drugs.

Perhaps most importantly, these examples reinforce the potential impact of performing DNA sequencing in tumor cells from patients with BPDCN. From a research perspective, there is likely still much more to be understood about BPDCN genetics. Clinically, DNA sequencing may identify mutated targets for treatment, particularly in the relapsed disease setting where current therapeutic options are limited.

Table 1
Active clinical trials currently recruiting patients with blastic plasmacytoid dendritic cell neoplasm

Agent	Phase	Key Eligibility	Clinicaltrials.gov ID#
Venetoclax	1	Relapsed disease or treatment-naïve but ineligible for standard therapy	NCT03485547
IMGN632 (anti-CD123 ADC)	1	Relapsed disease	NCT03386513
XmAb14045 (CD123 x CD3 bispecific T-cell engager)	1	Relapsed disease	NCT02730312
CD123 CAR T cell (autologous)	1	Relapsed disease	NCT02159495
Combination chemotherapy (idarubicin, methotrexate, L-asparaginase, dexamethasone) followed by stem cell transplantation	2	Treatment-naive	NCT03599960

Abbreviations: ADC, antibody-drug conjugate; CAR, chimeric antigen receptor.
Courtesy of the U.S. National Library of Medicine.

SUMMARY AND AREAS FOR IMPROVEMENT

The laboratory research and clinical trials that resulted in tagraxofusp becoming the first approved therapy for BPDCN have paved the way for additional studies in the disease. This article has outlined several targeted treatments that have promise, either as single agents, in combination with tagraxofusp, or as components of other novel combinations (see **Fig. 1**). Several of these drugs are already in trials for patients with BPDCN (**Table 1**).

The author's current approach to treatment is to give induction therapy, with tagraxofusp or an alternative regimen, and then proceed to stem cell transplantation if a complete remission is achieved. However, many additional questions remain unanswered. There are no standardized uniform response criteria for BPDCN trials, which makes comparing novel regimens challenging. Clinically, optimal salvage therapy for relapsed or refractory disease is not defined nor is the best approach for patients who do not undergo transplant. Also, no studies to date have examined the impact of maintenance therapy after achieving remission or after stem cell transplant. Nor have there been analyses of measurable residual disease (MRD) in BPDCN and its relationship to therapy selection or outcome. The new targeted approaches outlined here might be ideal candidates to test in the maintenance setting in addition to evaluation in patients with overt disease, particularly if they can be paired with MRD measurements. The author believes that BPDCN disease-specific laboratory and clinical research, rather than simply attaching to other leukemia studies, is the best path to continued improvement in patient outcomes.

ACKNOWLEDGMENTS

The author thanks Jacqueline Garcia for critical feedback on this article.

DISCLOSURE

A.A. Lane has received research support from AbbVie and Stemline Therapeutics and consulting fees from N-of-One/Qiagen.

REFERENCES

1. Khoury JD. Blasticplasmacytoid dendritic cell neoplasm. CurrHematolMalig Rep 2018;13:477–83.
2. Venugopal S, Zhou S, El Jamal SM, et al. Blasticplasmacytoid dendritic cell neoplasm-current insights. ClinLymphomaMyelomaLeuk 2019;19:545–54.
3. Sapienza MR, Pileri A, Derenzini E, et al. Blasticplasmacytoid dendritic cell neoplasm: state of the art and prospects. Cancers (Basel) 2019;11 [pii:E595].
4. Taylor J, Haddadin M, Upadhyay VA, et al. Multicenter analysis of outcomes in blasticplasmacytoid dendritic cell neoplasm offers a pretargeted therapy benchmark. Blood 2019;134:678–87.
5. Pagano L, Valentini CG, Pulsoni A, et al. Blasticplasmacytoid dendritic cell neoplasm with leukemic presentation: an Italian multicenter study. Haematologica 2013;98:239–46.
6. Syed YY. Tagraxofusp: first global approval. Drugs 2019;79:579–83.
7. Frankel AE, Woo JH, Ahn C, et al. Activity of SL-401, a targeted therapy directed to interleukin-3 receptor, in blasticplasmacytoid dendritic cell neoplasm patients. Blood 2014;124:385–92.
8. Economides MP, McCue D, Lane AA, et al. Tagraxofusp, the first CD123-targeted therapy and first targeted treatment for blasticplasmacytoid dendritic cell neoplasm. Expert Rev ClinPharmacol 2019;12(10):941–6.
9. Pemmaraju N, Lane AA, Sweet KL, et al. Tagraxofusp in blasticplasmacytoid dendritic-cell neoplasm. N Engl J Med 2019;380:1628–37.
10. Garnache-Ottou F, Feuillard J, Ferrand C, et al. Extended diagnostic criteria for plasmacytoid dendritic cell leukaemia. Br J Haematol 2009;145:624–36.
11. Dolgin E. First CD123-targeted drug approved after wowing in rare cancer. Nat Biotechnol 2019;37:202–3.
12. Kovtun Y, Jones GE, Adams S, et al. A CD123-targeting antibody-drug conjugate, IMGN632, designed to eradicate AML while sparing normal bone marrow cells. BloodAdv 2018;2:848–58.
13. Crossland DL, Denning WL, Ang S, et al. Antitumor activity of CD56-chimeric antigen receptor T cells in neuroblastoma and SCLC models. Oncogene 2018;37:3686–97.
14. John S, Chen H, Deng M, et al. A novel anti-LILRB4 CAR-T cell for the treatment of monocytic AML. MolTher 2018;26:2487–95.
15. Shah MH, Lorigan P, O'Brien ME, et al. Phase I study of IMGN901, a CD56-targeting antibody-drug conjugate, in patients with CD56-positive solid tumors. Invest NewDrugs 2016;34:290–9.
16. Leroux D, Mugneret F, Callanan M, et al. CD4(+), CD56(+) DC2 acute leukemia is characterized by recurrent clonal chromosomal changes affecting 6 major targets: a study of 21 cases by the GroupeFrancais de CytogenetiqueHematologique. Blood 2002;99:4154–9.
17. Dijkman R, van Doorn R, Szuhai K, et al. Gene-expression profiling and array-based CGH classify CD4+CD56+ hematodermic neoplasm and cutaneous myelomonocytic leukemia as distinct disease entities. Blood 2007;109:1720–7.
18. Lucioni M, Novara F, Fiandrino G, et al. Twenty-one cases of blasticplasmacytoid dendritic cell neoplasm: focus on biallelic locus 9p21.3 deletion. Blood 2011;118:4591–4.
19. Tang Z, Li Y, Wang W, et al. Genomic aberrations involving 12p/ETV6 are highly prevalent in blasticplasmacytoid dendritic cell neoplasms and might represent early clonal events. Leuk Res 2018;73:86–94.

20. Tang Z, Tang G, Wang SA, et al. Simultaneous deletion of 3′ETV6 and 5′EWSR1 genes in blasticplasmacytoid dendritic cell neoplasm: case report and literature review. MolCytogenet 2016;9:23.

21. Kubota S, Tokunaga K, Umezu T, et al. Lineage-specific RUNX2 super-enhancer activates MYC and promotes the development of blasticplasmacytoid dendritic cell neoplasm. Nat Commun 2019;10:1653.

22. Sakamoto K, Katayama R, Asaka R, et al. Recurrent 8q24 rearrangement in blasticplasmacytoid dendritic cell neoplasm: association with immunoblastoidcytomorphology, MYC expression, and drug response. Leukemia 2018;32:2590–603.

23. Suzuki K, Suzuki Y, Hama A, et al. Recurrent MYB rearrangement in blasticplasmacytoid dendritic cell neoplasm. Leukemia 2017;31:1629–33.

24. Sapienza MR, Abate F, Melle F, et al. Blasticplasmacytoid dendritic cell neoplasm: genomics mark epigenetic dysregulation as a primary therapeutic target. Haematologica 2019;104:729–37.

25. Menezes J, Acquadro F, Wiseman M, et al. Exome sequencing reveals novel and recurrent mutations with clinical impact in blasticplasmacytoid dendritic cell neoplasm. Leukemia 2014;28:823–9.

26. Stenzinger A, Endris V, Pfarr N, et al. Targeted ultra-deep sequencing reveals recurrent and mutually exclusive mutations of cancer genes in blasticplasmacytoid dendritic cell neoplasm. Oncotarget 2014;5:6404–13.

27. Sapienza MR, Fuligni F, Agostinelli C, et al. Molecular profiling of blasticplasmacytoid dendritic cell neoplasm reveals a unique pattern and suggests selective sensitivity to NF-kB pathway inhibition. Leukemia 2014;28:1606–16.

28. Montero J, Stephansky J, Cai T, et al. Blasticplasmacytoid dendritic cell neoplasm is dependent on BCL2 and sensitive to venetoclax. CancerDiscov 2017;7:156–64.

29. Del Gaizo Moore V, Letai A. BH3 profiling–measuring integrated function of the mitochondrial apoptotic pathway to predict cell fate decisions. CancerLett 2013;332:202–5.

30. Deng J, Carlson N, Takeyama K, et al. BH3 profiling identifies three distinct classes of apoptotic blocks to predict response to ABT-737 and conventional chemotherapeutic agents. Cancer Cell 2007;12:171–85.

31. Ryan J, Montero J, Rocco J, et al. iBH3: simple, fixable BH3 profiling to determine apoptotic priming in primary tissue by flow cytometry. BiolChem 2016;397:671–8.

32. Roberts AW, Davids MS, Pagel JM, et al. Targeting BCL2 with venetoclax in relapsed chronic lymphocytic leukemia. N Engl J Med 2016;374:311–22.

33. Carrington EM, Zhang JG, Sutherland RM, et al. ProsurvivalBcl-2 family members reveal a distinct apoptotic identity between conventional and plasmacytoid dendritic cells. ProcNatlAcadSciUS A 2015;112:4044–9.

34. Grushchak S, Joy C, Gray A, et al. Novel treatment of blasticplasmacytoid dendritic cell neoplasm: a case report. Medicine (Baltimore) 2017;96:e9452.

35. DiNardo CD, Rausch CR, Benton C, et al. Clinical experience with the BCL2-inhibitor venetoclax in combination therapy for relapsed and refractory acute myeloid leukemia and related myeloid malignancies. Am J Hematol 2018;93: 401–7.

36. Agha ME, Monaghan SA, Swerdlow SH. Venetoclax in a patient with a blasticplasmacytoid dendritic-cell neoplasm. N Engl J Med 2018;379:1479–81.

37. Pemmaraju N, Konopleva M, Lane AA. More on blasticplasmacytoid dendritic-cell neoplasms. N Engl J Med 2019;380:695–6.

38. Togami K, Pastika T, Stephansky J, et al. DNA methyltransferase inhibition overcomes diphthamide pathway deficiencies underlying CD123-targeted treatment resistance. J Clin Invest 2019;129(11):5005–19.

39. Bhojwani D, Sposto R, Shah NN, et al. Inotuzumabozogamicin in pediatric patients with relapsed/refractory acute lymphoblastic leukemia. Leukemia 2019; 33:884–92.

40. Ruella M, Maus MV. Catch me if you can: leukemia escape after CD19-Directed T Cell Immunotherapies. ComputStructBiotechnol J 2016;14:357–62.

41. Ceribelli M, Hou ZE, Kelly PN, et al. A druggableTCF4- and BRD4-dependent transcriptional network sustains malignancy in blasticplasmacytoid dendritic cell neoplasm. Cancer Cell 2016;30:764–78.

42. Su X, Lin Z, Lin H. The biosynthesis and biological function of diphthamide. Crit Rev BiochemMolBiol 2013;48:515–21.

43. Ni Chonghaile T, Sarosiek KA, Vo TT, et al. Pretreatment mitochondrial priming correlates with clinical response to cytotoxic chemotherapy. Science 2011;334: 1129–33.

44. Vo TT, Ryan J, Carrasco R, et al. Relative mitochondrial priming of myeloblasts and normal HSCs determines chemotherapeutic success in AML. Cell 2012; 151:344–55.

45. Khwaja R, Daly A, Wong M, et al. Azacitidine in the treatment of blasticplasmacytoid dendritic cell neoplasm: a report of 3 cases. LeukLymphoma 2016;57: 2720–2.

46. Laribi K, Denizon N, Ghnaya H, et al. Blasticplasmacytoid dendritic cell neoplasm: the first report of two cases treated by 5-azacytidine. Eur J Haematol 2014;93:81–5.

47. Ghosh HS, Cisse B, Bunin A, et al. Continuous expression of the transcription factor e2-2 maintains the cell fate of mature plasmacytoid dendritic cells. Immunity 2010;33:905–16.

48. Grajkowska LT, Ceribelli M, Lau CM, et al. Isoform-specific expression and feedback regulation of E protein TCF4control dendritic cell lineage specification. Immunity 2017;46:65–77.

49. Shi J, Vakoc CR. The mechanisms behind the therapeutic activity of BET bromodomain inhibition. MolCell 2014;54:728–36.

50. Emadali A, Hoghoughi N, Duley S, et al. Haploinsufficiency for NR3C1, the gene encoding the glucocorticoid receptor, in blasticplasmacytoid dendritic cell neoplasms. Blood 2016;127:3040–53.

51. Ceroi A, Masson D, Roggy A, et al. LXR agonist treatment of blasticplasmacytoid dendritic cell neoplasm restores cholesterol efflux and triggers apoptosis. Blood 2016;128:2694–707.

52. Wang B, Tontonoz P. Liver X receptors in lipid signalling and membrane homeostasis. Nat Rev Endocrinol 2018;14:452–63.

53. Boddu PC, Wang SA, Pemmaraju N, et al. 8q24/MYC rearrangement is a recurrent cytogenetic abnormality in blasticplasmacytoid dendritic cell neoplasms. Leuk Res 2018;66:73–8.

54. Ramaswamy K, Forbes L, Minuesa G, et al. Peptidomimetic blockade of MYB in acute myeloid leukemia. Nat Commun 2018;9:110.

55. Philippe L, Ceroi A, Bole-Richard E, et al. Bortezomib as a new therapeutic approach for blasticplasmacytoid dendritic cell neoplasm. Haematologica 2017;102:1861–8.

56. Agliano A, Martin-Padura I, Marighetti P, et al. Therapeutic effect of lenalidomide in a novel xenograft mouse model of human blasticNK cell lymphoma/blasticplasmacytoid dendritic cell neoplasm. ClinCancer Res 2011;17:6163–73.

57. Marmouset V, Joris M, Merlusca L, et al. The lenalidomide/bortezomib/dexamethasone regimen for the treatment of blasticplasmacytoid dendritic cell neoplasm. HematolOncol 2019;37(4):487–9.

58. Yang C, Fu C, Feng Y, et al. Clinical efficacy of bortezomib and lenalidomide in blasticplasmacytoid dendritic cell neoplasm. Ann Hematol 2019;98:1525–7.

59. Riaz W, Zhang L, Horna P, et al. Blasticplasmacytoid dendritic cell neoplasm: update on molecular biology, diagnosis, and therapy. Cancer Control 2014;21: 279–89.

60. Norsworthy KJ, Luo L, Hsu V, et al. FDA approval summary: ivosidenib for relapsed or refractory acute myeloid leukemia with an isocitrate dehydrogenase-1 mutation. ClinCancer Res 2019;25:3205–9.

61. Dugan J, Pollyea D. Enasidenib for the treatment of acute myeloid leukemia. Expert Rev ClinPharmacol 2018;11:755–60.

62. Perl AE. Availability of FLT3 inhibitors: how do we use them? Blood 2019;134: 741–5.

63. Lee SC, Dvinge H, Kim E, et al. Modulation of splicing catalysis for therapeutic targeting of leukemia with mutations in genes encoding spliceosomal proteins. Nat Med 2016;22:672–8.

Blastic Plasmacytoid Dendritic Cell Neoplasm in Children

Yixian Li, MD[a], Victoria Sun, PhD[b], Weili Sun, MD, PhD[b,c],
Anna Pawlowska, MD[b,*]

KEYWORDS

- Pediatric blastic plasmacytoid dendritic cell neoplasm • CD123 • CD4 • leukemia
- Stem cell transplant • Tagraxofusp

KEY POINTS

- Blastic plasmacytoid dendritic cell neoplasm (BPDCN) is an extremely rare type of neoplasm seen in adult and pediatric patients.
- Focal positivity of S-100 in neoplastic cells occurs at a higher frequency in pediatric populations, along with other markers of plasmacytoid dendritic cells.
- Acute lymphoid leukemia/Acute myeloid leukemia/lymphoma-type chemotherapy has been used to treat pediatric BPDCN, both with and without stem cell transplant. Currently, high-risk acute lymphoblastic leukemia therapy regimens with central nervous system prophylaxis are recommended.
- Stem cell transplant in pediatric patients may be reserved for relapsed/refractory disease or high-risk disease at presentation.
- Targeted therapy using the anti-CD123 (interleukin-3 receptor) immunotoxin tagraxofusp has been approved by the US Food and Drug Administration for children more than 2 years of age. Incorporation of the drug into chemotherapy, and its role as a bridge to transplant, remains unclear.

INTRODUCTION

Blastic plasmacytoid dendritic cell neoplasm (BPDCN) is a rare, clinically aggressive hematological malignancy derived from a unique dendritic cell subset called plasmacytoid dendritic cells (pDCs), or type 2 dendritic cells.[1–3] It is typically characterized by involvement of the skin (dermatopathic) and/or peripheral blood and bone marrow.

[a] Pediatric Hematology, Oncology, Marrow and Blood Cell Transplantation, Children's Hospital at Montefiore, 3411 Wayne Avenue, 9th Floor, Bronx, NY 10467, USA; [b] Pediatric Hematology, Oncology and Hematopoietic Stem Cell Transplantation, City of Hope, 1500 East Duarte Road, Duarte, CA 91010, USA; [c] Janssen Pharmaceuticals, 10990 Wilshire Boulevard, Suite 300, Los Angeles, CA 90024, USA
* Corresponding author.
E-mail address: apawlowska@coh.org

Hematol Oncol Clin N Am 34 (2020) 601–612
https://doi.org/10.1016/j.hoc.2020.01.008
0889-8588/20/© 2020 Elsevier Inc. All rights reserved.

Although predominantly affecting older adults with a median age of 65 years, rare cases of BPDCN have been reported across all age groups, including infants and children. Pediatric BPDCN has been more widely recognized and reported since the World Health Organization (WHO) established diagnostic criteria in 2008.[3,4]

BPDCN was initially described in a 1994 case report from Japan as a cluster of differentiation (CD) 4–positive cutaneous lymphoma with high CD56 expression.[5] It was later concluded that the clinical features of CD4+/CD56+ malignancies corresponded to pDCs.[6] However, the diagnostic criteria of BPDCN were not clearly defined until the 2008 WHO Classification of Tumors of Hematopoietic and Lymphoid Tissues recognized it as a distinct clinicopathologic entity. Experiences treating children with BPDCN have been rare, with limited reports in the literature.

A case study conducted at the National Cancer Institute (NCI) in 2010 evaluated BPDCN outcomes in children both within the National Institutes of Health (NIH) and across the literature with ages ranging from less than 1 year to 18 years. The investigators concluded that pediatric BPDCN is clinically less aggressive, and often associated with a more favorable outcome when treated with high-risk acute lymphoblastic leukemia (ALL) chemotherapy and central nervous system (CNS) prophylaxis. Furthermore, the investigators recommended reserving stem cell transplant (SCT) in children for the following cases: (1) second complete remission (CR), or (2) when initial treatment does not induce a rapid or complete remission.[1,3] Outcomes from this study and several others highlighting pediatric cases of BPDCN are summarized and discussed in this article.

To date, ALL/acute myeloid leukemia (AML)/non-Hodgkin lymphoma (NHL)–type chemotherapy regimens have been used to treat patients with BPDCN. In adults, treatment is typically followed by SCT because of the aggressiveness of disease and poor outcomes.[7,8] However, for pediatric populations, some experts recommend observation after first remission because of more favorable outcomes, reserving transplant for children who relapse and achieve a second remission.[3] However, although this remains one of the most comprehensive studies on pediatric BPDCN outcomes, the analysis was performed on only 29 children and larger studies are necessary in order to determine the role of SCT for younger populations.[3,9]

Recently, a novel targeted therapy, tagraxofusp (a CD123-directed cytotoxin), showed improved overall response rate in a clinical trial involving adult patients with untreated or relapsed BPDCN.[10] In a case report including 3 pediatric patients with BPDCN, tagraxofusp showed encouraging, although transient, clinical responses.[11] Based on these results, tagraxofusp has been indicated for use in pediatric patients, and, in December 2019, was approved in the United States by the Food and Drug Administration (FDA) for adults and children 2 years of age and older.[11,12]

PATHOPHYSIOLOGIC AND PATHOLOGIC FEATURES

Previously named blastic natural killer (NK) cell leukemia/lymphoma, based on the blastic appearance and CD56 expression, BPDCN is understood to originate from pDC precursors.[1,6,13] pDCs are a subtype of immune cells distinguished by their capacity to secrete large quantities of type 1 interferon (IFNs) in response to a viral infection. They have secretory plasma cell–like morphology and express several surface antigens important in the role of linking the innate and adaptive immune systems.[14,15]

Molecular profiling on an extensive panel of samples (n = 25) performed by Sapienza and colleagues[16] defined the cellular counterpart and confirmed the nuclear factor kappa B (NF-κB) pathway activation in BPDCNs. Details on the cell of origin and pathogenesis of BPDCN based on gene expression profiling can be found in other articles in this issue. Briefly, by comparing the BPDCN samples with normal pDC samples isolated from healthy donors as a control, the cellular derivation of BPDCN was proved to originate from the myeloid lineage and, in particular, from resting pDCs. Further, the investigators' study validating the effectiveness of NF-κB pathway inhibitors ex vivo provided the first rationale for a molecular-targeted therapy. Similar studies evaluating gene expression profiles and assessing the NF-κB pathway as a candidate therapeutic target have not been performed on pediatric samples.

Morphologically, BPDCN presents with monomorphic, agranular, medium-sized blast cells in affected tissue (most commonly skin, followed by lymph nodes and spleen) and/or peripheral blood/bone marrow. The blast cells are often lymphoblast-like, with condensed chromatin and scant cytoplasm, and are occasionally myeloblastlike, with larger dispersed chromatin and more adequate cytoplasm. Two unique but nonspecific findings are a pseudopod cytoplasm extension and circumferential cytoplasmic microvacuoles (pearl-necklace appearance).[17] Although the cause of discrepancy in clinical behavior between adult and pediatric patients remains uncertain, histologic differences between the two populations have been documented.[3,18] In a series of 25 specimens collected from adult patients with BPDCN, tumor cells revealed a pleomorphic appearance containing blastoid cells with elongated, twisted, or hyperchromatic cells, as opposed to the fairly uniform and lymphoblastlike appearance of neoplastic cells among pediatric patients studied.

Immunophenotypes can be diagnostic features for BPDCN, either by immunohistochemistry or flow cytometry. The classic immunophenotypic profile for BPDCN is positive for CD4, CD56, CD45RA, and HLA-DR (human leukocyte antigen, DR isotype), and the pDC-associated antigens CD123 (interleukin-3 receptor), TCL1A (T-cell leukemia/lymphoma-1), CD303 (BDCA-2 [blood dendritic cell antigen-2]), and CD2AP, and negative for CD3, CD13, CD16, CD19, CD20, CD34, myeloperoxidase (MPO), CD117, lysozyme, and Epstein-Barr virus–encoded small RNA (EBER).[2,7,17] Some patients show expression of CD2, CD5, CD7, CD117, and terminal deoxynucleotidyl transferase (TdT).[1,19] CD123, a highly expressed membrane marker, has been explored as a potential diagnostic and therapeutic target for BPDCN.

Rarely, CD56-negative cases have been reported, and a diagnosis can be made with other characteristic markers, particularly pDC-associated markers. No specific cytogenetic mutations have been reported.[2,7,20–22] Further, the functional significance of S-100 expression, a family of genes expressing damage-associated molecular patterns molecules, may be of potential interest, especially for pediatric patients. In a 2009 review published by the NIH, focal positivity of S-100 in neoplastic cells was detected in 75% of pediatric patients (3 of 4), as opposed to only 25% of adult patients (5 of 20) tested.[3] Given the rarity of BPDCN, these observations come from a small number of patients but may provide insight in defining prognostic markers in the future.

A 2017 study including 14 patients with BPDCN (5 children, 9 adults) identified recurring MYB gene rearrangements to occur at a higher frequency in children (100%) than in adults (44%).[23] The MYB protein is a DNA-binding transcription factor, and is understood to be one of the key regulators of vertebrate hematopoiesis.[24,25] Abnormalities in the MYB locus have been identified across several hematopoietic cell lines and primary hematological malignancies, and their direct involvement in human leukemia has been widely explored.[25] Further, these have been found to be associated with several pediatric disease subtypes, including childhood myeloid leukemias,[26] pediatric T-cell ALL,[27] and infant acute basophilic leukemia.[28] In the 2017 study, gene set enrichment analysis conducted with publicly available expression data[16] confirmed the upregulation of MYB downstream target genes in younger patients.[23] Although the findings from this study involve a small patient sample (n = 14), they provide evidence that MYB translocations or other MYB-activating events occur at a higher frequency among younger patients, and identify the proto-oncogene as a potential diagnostic marker and molecular therapeutic target in pediatric BPDCN.

CLINICAL PRESENTATIONS

BPDCN is widely considered a CD4+/CD56+ hematodermic neoplasm/tumor, because of its proclivity for cutaneous involvement. Most patients (80%–85%) present with skin lesions, which may be either localized or widespread, and vary from subtle, bruiselike macules to purplish plaques, nodules, or tumors.[15] Isolated skin lesions are more often located on the head or lower extremities and can spread to multiple locations and become disseminated. A subset of patients presents with more diffuse disease. Examining physicians should be alerted to the possibility of BPDCN when the diffuse presentation of nodules and patches is observed.[17]

Other commonly involved sites include bone marrow or peripheral blood, and any tissue type may be infiltrated, ranging from lymph nodes and the spleen to rarer tissues, including the nasopharynx, uterus, and ovaries. Similar to other types of leukemia, CNS involvement with BPDCN is common. In a subgroup analysis of pediatric patients whose CNS status was known, a higher rate of involvement of tumors or tumor cells in the brain, spinal cord, or cerebrospinal fluid was indicated.[29] Leukocytosis and cytopenia of other lineages are also common (especially thrombocytopenia).[2,3,7] Nonspecific symptoms associated with BPDCN include fever, pallor, lymphadenopathy, and hepatosplenomegaly. In most cases, if the disease is not controlled early or at onset, the disseminated leukemic phase will ultimately develop.

Although cutaneous involvement may be more common among pediatric patients than previously reported in adults, for the minority of patients lacking cutaneous disease at presentation, more favorable outcomes have anecdotally been indicated. A 2013 review of literature including 32 pediatric patients evaluated overall survival for children presenting with versus without cutaneous disease.[9] The overall survival in patients with skin involvement was 40.5% ± 13.6% (24 patients), with 6 of 23 patients receiving allogeneic SCT in first or second remission. Remarkably, the overall survival in patients who lacked skin involvement was 100% (8 patients), with 2 of 8 patients receiving allogeneic SCT in first or second remission. Although statistically significant, the number of cases is too small to make any definitive conclusions. However, the study results suggest less aggressive disease when children with BPDCN present without skin involvement.

DIAGNOSIS AND DIFFERENTIAL DIAGNOSIS

The diagnosis of BPDCN is heavily dependent on microscopic morphology and immunophenotyping, particularly for patients presenting with nonspecific dermatologic lesions. Importantly, none of the antigens constituting the typical immunophenotypic profile may be used individually as a diagnostic tool, because many of these markers may be present in other cell types and diseases.[17] Thus, thorough cytologic and immunophenotypic evaluation is required to exclude common mimickers of the BPDCN profile. Morphologic review is useful, but can be difficult; studies including gene expression profiling possess the potential to provide further insight into the pathobiology of the disease. A typical immunophenotype profile with positive CD4, CD56, CD123, CD303, and TCL1A, and negative CD3, CD13, CD16, CD19, CD20, lysozyme, and MPO are reliable tools for diagnosing BPDCN.[1,3,7,17]

Differential Diagnosis

Differential diagnostic considerations for BPDCN range from acute leukemia, myeloid and lymphoid types, and myeloid sarcoma/leukemia cutis to NK/T-cell lymphoma/leukemia, blastic mantle cell lymphoma, and other high-grade lymphomas, to chronic myeloid malignancies.[2,7,17] A detailed investigation of cytologic and/or immunophenotypic similarities across the literature was published in 2013.[17] Many of the markers positive in BPDCN are not individually specific for establishing a diagnosis, and immunophenotypic overlap of these markers may be seen with non-BPDCN entities. The most challenging in the differential diagnosis include:

1. AML/monocytic leukemia and myeloid sarcoma/myeloid leukemia cutis: BPDCN can present with circulating blasts, morphologically resembling myeloid blasts. AML shares some immunophenotyping with BPDCN, including CD123, CD56, and sometimes CD33. Importantly, the 2010 NCI study reported that none of the 28 patients with AML expressed S-100.[3]
2. NK/T-cell leukemia/lymphoma: positive for CD2 and CD56, but associated with Epstein-Barr virus infection and can be positive for EBER.
3. Mature plasmacytoid dendritic cell proliferation: can be associated with cutaneous lesions and lymph node/bone marrow involvement. The pDCs are morphologically mature and CD56 negative.

TREATMENT

There is no universal consensus for the treatment of BPDCN in children, because of rarity and a considerable absence of prospective clinical trials. The therapy regimens in adults typically consist of ALL/AML/lymphomalike chemotherapy, whereas the ALL-like regimen yielded better overall survival outcomes, followed by allogeneic SCT.[3,8,30] However, the treatment regimen in children varies, depending on physician experience and patient response to chemotherapy.

The current recommendation for treatment (high-risk ALL therapy with CNS prophylaxis, reserving SCT for second CR) is based on the 2010 NCI retrospective study, which analyzed overall survival rates in 29 cases of BPDCN presenting in patients less than the age of 18 years.[3] Of the 29 cases, 9 were reviewed at the NIH, whereas 20 were identified in the literature. Immunohistochemical studies, flow cytometry, and cytogenetic results were reported, and all 29 patients were positive for CD4 and all but one case was positive for CD56. CD123, excluding 8 cases for which staining was not determined, were all positive. Furthermore, CD68 was negative in all but one case, which showed focal punctate staining.[3]

Clinical follow-up was available for 25 of 29 patients, with follow-up ranging between 9 months and 13 years, and all patients received chemotherapy. The overall survival rate among the 25 patients was 72%, and the event-free survival (EFS) rate was 64%. Fourteen patients in the series initially received ALL-type therapy regimens, with 12 achieving remission and 2 achieving partial response (PR). Two of those patients underwent SCT, 1 in first CR and 1 in second CR,[6,31] and both were reported to be disease free at their last follow-up. There was only 1 reported death in the ALL-type therapy group without SCT; this occurred in a child with cutaneous involvement at presentation and relatively advanced disease.

Treatment with other forms of chemotherapy was also reported. Four of 6 patients treated with NHL-type therapy survived, with 3 undergoing SCT, 1 in first CR, 1 in first CR after receiving ALL-type therapy, and 1 in second CR after receiving ALL therapy.[32–35] Because BPDCN is no longer considered to be a lymphoma, instead representing a unique precursor hematopoietic neoplasm, it is not considered curable with treatment regimens for NHL.[15] Notably, AML-type therapy was limited to 3 cases, and all 3 patients died, 1 of progressive disease and 2 of therapy-related complications.[6,36,37]

In a smaller study conducted in 2013 at St. Jude Children's Research Hospital, investigators reported 4 pediatric patients between the ages of 6 and 11 years who were treated with their institutional ALL protocol and remained in CR without SCT.[4] Three of the 4 patients completed treatment, remaining in continuous CR 5.8 years, 4.2 years, and 11.1 years from diagnosis, respectively, as of 2013. The fourth patient remained in remission after induction chemotherapy and surgical resection, but was lost to follow-up after transferring care. The successful results reported in this study support arguments in favor of an intensive ALL-based regimen for pediatric patients with dendritic cell leukemia.

The impact of initial sites of involvement and treatment modalities on outcome has been summarized previously for the 29 pediatric cases detailed in the 2010 NCI study.[3] Briefly, a majority of the patients (22 of 29, 76%) had skin involvement, and the remaining 7 (24%) lacked cutaneous disease at presentation. Those 7 with disease confined to the bone marrow, peripheral blood, lymph nodes, spleen, and/or liver, in addition to 8/29 patients presenting with initial cutaneous disease, all received ALL-type chemotherapy regimens. All patients lacking cutaneous disease at presentation were alive at a median follow-up of 60 months (7 of 7, 100%), and only 2 of the 8 patients with initial cutaneous disease died. Among the 18 patients who presented with cutaneous disease and for whom follow-up data were available, only 11 survived (61%). Results indicating an improved overall survival in patients without skin involvement at presentation have been corroborated by subsequent experiences at additional institutions.[9,38] However, more studies are needed to determine the prognostic significance of cutaneous involvement.

Contrary to that for the adult population, the current recommendation suggests ALL-type chemotherapy followed by observation, rather than allogeneic SCT, in first remission for pediatric patients with BPDCN. In the 2010 NCI study of pediatric patients with BPDCN, the investigators compared overall survival rates between patients who underwent transplant and those who did not. For patients who did not undergo transplant, the overall survival was 74% (14 of 19 patients). In contrast, the overall survival of all pediatric patients who underwent transplant was 67% (4 of 6 patients), with 2 of the survivors transplanted in second remission. Of the 2 posttransplant deaths, 1 was attributed to transplant-related complications and the other was disease related. Thus, for children who achieve CR, the present consensus regarding transplant suggests that the toxicity of allogeneic SCT in first remission outweighs the potential improvement of longer-term outcomes.

A novel CD123-directed cytotoxin, tagraxofusp (SL-401), was approved by the FDA in 2018 for the treatment of patients with BPDCN aged 2 years and older.[12] In vitro, it was shown to have significantly higher cytotoxicity than cytarabine, cyclophosphamide, vincristine, dexamethasone, methotrexate, Erwinia L-asparaginase, or asparaginase in primary BPDCN cells.[38] In a study including 47 adult patients, the overall response rate (PR rate or better) was 90% (29 patients) for previously untreated patients and 67% (15 patients) for previously treated patients.[10] Thirteen of the 29 previously untreated patients (45%) were successfully bridged to SCT while in remission after tagraxofusp. One of the 15 previously treated patients who had disease remission while receiving tagraxofusp underwent allogeneic SCT.

To our knowledge, a clinical trial evaluating the safety and efficacy of tagraxofusp in children with BPDCN has never been conducted. In the first reported pediatric experience, Sun and colleagues[11] showed the feasibility of using the CD123-targeted therapy to treat pediatric BPDCN, through compassionate use. Three patients between the ages of 10 and 15 years were administered the adult dosing regimen for tagraxofusp, receiving a 5-day infusion of 12 µg/kg/d every 2 to 3 weeks. Overall, the treatment was well tolerated with minimal toxicities and side effects similar to those observed in adult patients, including capillary leak syndrome and infusion reaction.[39] One patient with multiple relapsed and refractory disease had no response. The other 2 patients showed significant and rapid clinical improvement after 2 courses of treatment, as indicated by **Fig. 1**. After 2 courses of treatment, the soft tissue mass of patient #2 had decreased significantly in size. Considerable responses in bone marrow CD123 staining, showing a decrease in circulating blasts as well as marked improvement of pulmonary lymphadenopathy, was seen in patient #3. However, the positive response was transient. After 2 to 3 months of treatment, both patients showed evidence of disease progression.

Investigational therapies, although primarily reported in adult populations, include B-cell lymphoma 2 (BCL-2) inhibitors,[40–43] chimeric antigen receptor T-cell therapy,[43] hypomethylating therapy,[44–46] bromodomain inhibition,[47–50] and NF-κB pathway inhibitors.[16,51] The clinical activity of such therapies in BPDCN has previously been summarized[52] and is discussed in other articles in this issue. The potential benefit of these therapies remains an important research question, but a high-risk ALL-type regimen remains the recommended first-line treatment of pediatric patients.

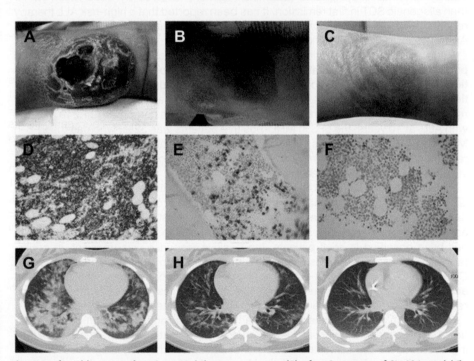

Fig. 1. Left ankle mass of patient #2 (A) pretreatment, (B) after 2 courses of SL-401, and (C) after hematopoietic cell transplant. (D, G) Bone marrow CD123 staining and chest computed tomography of patient #3 pretreatment, (E, H) after 1 course of SL-401, and (F, I) after 2 courses of SL-401. (From Sun W, Liu H, Kim Y, et al. First pediatric experience of SL-401, a CD123-targeted therapy, in patients with blastic plasmacytoid dendritic cell neoplasm: report of three cases. J Hematol Oncol 2018;11(1):61; with permission.)

DISCUSSION

BPDCN is a rare, aggressive neoplasm arising from precursors of the type 2 dendritic cells or pDCs. An accurate diagnosis requires biopsy and morphologic assessment of the involved tissue, and proper evaluation of histology and immunophenotyping remains heavily reliant on the expertise of a dermatopathologist /hematopathologist. An immunophenotypic panel of CD4, CD56, CD123, TCL1A, and CD303 positivity is almost diagnostic, with the negative biomarkers to rule out myeloid, lymphoblastic, and NK cell lineages. Although rare, a minority of CD4-negative or CD56-negative neoplasms can be seen if pDC-associated antigens CD123, TCL1A, or CD303 are positive.[2,7,17,53] Interestingly, a difference in S-100 expression has been noted between pediatric (75%) and adult (25%) patients reviewed at the NIH.[3]

The clinical features of BPDCN are largely attributable to the manifestation of dermatologic or leukemic presentations. Pediatric patients presenting with cutaneous involvement (85%) should be considered to have more aggressive disease, especially in patients with diffuse presentation of nodules, patches/plaques, and/or bruiselike lesions. For a minority of patients lacking skin involvement, those reported in the literature have a higher overall survival. However, the number of patients evaluated remains too small to make a definitive conclusion.

Treatment recommendations for pediatric BPDCN differ slightly from those for the adult population. For children with BPDCN, experts recommend therapy with an ALL/Lymphoblastic Lymphoma (LBL)-like regimen, followed by observation rather than allogeneic SCT in first remission. It has been reported that a high-risk ALL therapy regimen may produce a more favorable outcome in the pediatric population than AML-type or NHL-type chemotherapies.[3,4]

Pediatric patients presenting with very-high-risk disease, including patients with persistent disease or minimal residual disease (MRD) positivity in the end of induction/consolidation therapy, could be considered SCT candidates in first remission. Patients with a diagnosis of ALL with MRD positivity are at very high risk of disease recurrence. In a 2017 meta-analysis of 20 pediatric studies comprising 11,249 patients with ALL, at 10 years, the EFS in MRD-positive patients was 32%, whereas the EFS in MRD-negative patients was 77%.[54] Given that pediatric patients with BPDCN respond well to ALL-type therapy, results from this study could be considered by physicians in guiding ongoing treatment and SCT referral.

Targeted therapy using the CD123-directed immunotoxin tagraxofusp shows promising clinical responses and has been indicated for use in children. To date, only 3 patients receiving tagraxofusp have been reported in the literature, with acceptable toxicity and positive clinical responses seen in 2 of the 3 patients.[11] However, similar to what has been observed in adult patients, the positive response was transient. In adults, tagraxofusp has been used as a first-line therapy for treatment-naive patients because CR rates showed acceptable outcomes. However, most pediatric patients are able to achieve CR using ALL-type therapy, with tolerable toxicities. Thus, an ALL-type therapy remains the current recommendation as a first-line treatment of pediatric BPDCN.

Given the minimal toxicities and transient positive responses seen in pediatric patients, it is reasonable to consider tagraxofusp in combination with chemotherapy during consolidation or maintenance therapy for patients with newly diagnosed BPDCN. Implementing carefully designed clinical trials and comparing the results with historical data is required, because the small number of pediatric patients makes it unfeasible to design randomized trials. For patients with high-risk disease (eg, MRD positive), or patients in second CR, tagraxofusp is an optimal therapy to decrease MRD and bridge to SCT.

Although the toxicity of allogeneic SCT in first remission seemingly outweighs the potential improvement of longer-term outcomes, the role of transplant in subsequent relapsed/refractory disease is currently being explored. For relapsed or refractory BPDCN, treatment choice is determined by prior therapy, but participation in a clinical trial is favored. Beyond enrollment in clinical trials, an optimal treatment of patients who were previously treated with an ALL/LBL-like regimen may be salvage therapy with tagraxofusp, followed by allogeneic SCT.

After its recognition as an independent entity by the 2008 WHO classification, there have been more case series and reports of BPDCN, mainly in the adult population. However, the case reports and treatment experience in children remain extremely rare and multicentered, and prospective clinical trials are lacking.[3,6,8] Increasing awareness of pediatric BPDCN and understanding of the molecular basis, as well as reporting clinical case presentations, should lead to more accurate diagnoses and, ultimately, establish a standardized therapeutic approach.

The potential benefit of transplant and targeted therapies remains an important research question that should be studied in prospective clinical trials. At present, a multi-center retrospective study on pediatric BPDCN treatment outcomes has been approved by the Institutional Review Board and will be performed by investigators at City of Hope. The study, led by Dr Anna Pawlowska, will collect clinical information regarding disease characteristics, presentation, treatment, response, and survival across major pediatric oncology centers in the United States and globally. The database accrued from this study will serve as a platform to guide the design of future effective treatments.

DISCLOSURE

The authors have nothing to disclose.

REFERENCES

1. Facchetti F, JD, Petrella T. Blastic plasmacytoid dendritic cell neoplasm. In: Bosman FT, JE, Lakhani SR, et al, editors. WHO classification of tumours of hae-matopoietic and lymphoid tissues. Lyon (France): IARC Press; 2008. p. 145–7.

2. Facchetti F, PT, Pileri SA. Blastic plasmacytoid dendritic cell neoplasm. In: Bosman FT, JE, Lakhani SR, et al, editors. WHO classification of tumours of hae-matopoietic and lymphoid tissues. 4th (revised) edition. Lyon (France): IARC Press; 2016. p. 174–7.

3. Jegalian AG, Buxbaum NP, Facchetti F, et al. Blastic plasmacytoid dendritic cell neoplasm in children: diagnostic features and clinical implications. Haematolog-ica 2010;95(11):1873–9.

4. Wright KD, Onciu MM, Coustan Smith E, et al. Successful treatment of pediatric plasmacytoid dendritic cell tumors with a contemporary regimen for acute lymphoblastic leukemia. Pediatr Blood Cancer 2013;60(7):E38–41.

5. Adachi M, Maeda K, Takekawa M, et al. High expression of CD56 (NCAM) in a patient with cutaneous CD4-positive lymphoma. Am J Hematol 1994;47(4): 278–82.

6. Feuillard J, Jacob M-C, Valensi F, et al. Clinical and biologic features of CD4+ CD56+ malignancies. Blood 2002;99(5):1556–63.

7. Gurbuxani S. Blastic plasmacytoid dendritic cell neoplasm. Waltham (MA): UpTo-Date Inc; 2019. Last reviewed Aug 2019.

8. Trottier AM, Cerquozzi S, Owen CJ. Blastic plasmacytoid dendritic cell neoplasm: challenges and future prospects. Blood Lymphat Cancer 2017;7:85.

9. Sakashita K, Saito S, Yanagisawa R, et al. Usefulness of allogeneic hematopoietic stem cell transplantation in first complete remission for pediatric blastic plasmacytoid dendritic cell neoplasm with skin involvement: a case report and review of literature. Pediatr Blood Cancer 2013;60(11):E140–2.

10. Pemmaraju N, Lane AA, Sweet KL, et al. Tagraxofusp in blastic plasmacytoid dendritic-cell neoplasm. N Engl J Med 2019;380(17):1628–37.

11. Sun W, Liu H, Kim Y, et al. First pediatric experience of SL-401, a CD123-targeted therapy, in patients with blastic plasmacytoid dendritic cell neoplasm: report of three cases. J Hematol Oncol 2018;11(1):61.

12. Syed YY. Tagraxofusp: first global approval. Drugs 2019;79(5):579–83.

13. Chaperot L, Bendriss N, Manches O, et al. Identification of a leukemic counterpart of the plasmacytoid dendritic cells. Blood 2001;97(10):3210–7.

14. Reizis B, Bunin A, Ghosh HS, et al. Plasmacytoid dendritic cells: recent progress and open questions. Annu Rev Immunol 2011;29:163–83.

15. Jegalian AG, Facchetti F, Jaffe ES. Plasmacytoid dendritic cells: physiologic roles and pathologic states. Adv Anat Pathol 2009;16(6):392.

16. Sapienza M, Fuligni F, Agostinelli C, et al. Molecular profiling of blastic plasmacytoid dendritic cell neoplasm reveals a unique pattern and suggests selective sensitivity to NF-kB pathway inhibition. Leukemia 2014;28(8):1606.

17. Reichard KK. Blastic plasmacytoid dendritic cell neoplasm: how do you distinguish it from acute myeloid leukemia? Surg Pathol Clin 2013;6(4):743–65.

18. Cota C, Vale E, Viana I, et al. Cutaneous manifestations of blastic plasmacytoid dendritic cell neoplasm—morphologic and phenotypic variability in a series of 33 patients. Am J Surg Pathol 2010;34(1):75–87.

19. Pennisi M, Cesana C, Cittone MG, et al. A case of blastic plasmacytoid dendritic cell neoplasm extensively studied by flow cytometry and immunohistochemistry. Case Rep Hematol 2017;2017:4984951.

20. Garnache Ottou F, Feuillard J, Ferrand C, et al. Extended diagnostic criteria for plasmacytoid dendritic cell leukaemia. Br J Haematol 2009;145(5):624–36.

21. Testa U, Pelosi E, Frankel A. CD 123 is a membrane biomarker and a therapeutic target in hematologic malignancies. Biomark Res 2014;2(1):4.

22. Julia F, Dalle S, Duru G, et al. Blastic plasmacytoid dendritic cell neoplasms: clinico-immunohistochemical correlations in a series of 91 patients. Am J Surg Pathol 2014;38(5):673–80.

23. Suzuki K, Suzuki Y, Hama A, et al. Recurrent MYB rearrangement in blastic plasmacytoid dendritic cell neoplasm. Leukemia 2017;31(7):1629.

24. Soza-Ried C, Hess I, Netuschil N, et al. Essential role of c-myb in definitive hematopoiesis is evolutionarily conserved. Proc Natl Acad Sci U S A 2010;107(40):17304–8.

25. Pattabiraman D, Gonda T. Role and potential for therapeutic targeting of MYB in leukemia. Leukemia 2013;27(2):269.

26. Rosson D, Tereba A. Transcription of hematopoietic-associated oncogenes in childhood leukemia. Cancer Res 1983;43(8):3912–8.

27. Sinclair P, Harrison CJ, Jarosová M, et al. Analysis of balanced rearrangements of chromosome 6 in acute leukemia: clustered breakpoints in q22-q23 and possible involvement of c-MYB in a new recurrent translocation, t (6; 7)(q23; q32 through 36). Haematologica 2005;90(5):602–11.

28. Quelen C, Lippert E, Struski S, et al. Identification of a transforming MYB-GATA1 fusion gene in acute basophilic leukemia: a new entity in male infants. Blood 2011;117(21):5719–22.

29. Kim MJ, Nasr A, Kabir B, et al. Pediatric blastic plasmacytoid dendritic cell neoplasm: a systematic literature review. J Pediatr Hematol Oncol 2017;39(7): 528–37.

30. Piccaluga PP, Paolini S, Sapienza MR, et al. Blastic plasmacytoid dendritic cell neoplasm: is it time to redefine the standard of care? Expert Rev Hematol 2012;5(4):353–5.

31. Rossi JG, Felice MS, Bernasconi AR, et al. Acute leukemia of dendritic cell lineage in childhood: incidence, biological characteristics and outcome. Leuk Lymphoma 2006;47(4):715–25.

32. Shaw PH, Cohn SL, Morgan ER, et al. Natural killer cell lymphoma: report of two pediatric cases, therapeutic options, and review of the literature. Cancer 2001; 91(4):642–6.

33. Karube K, Ohshima K, Tsuchiya T, et al. Non-B, non-T neoplasms with lymphoblast morphology: further clarification and classification. Am J Surg Pathol 2003;27(10):1366–74.

34. Ruggiero A, Maurizi P, Larocca LM, et al. Childhood CD4+/CD56+ hematodermic neoplasm: case report and review of the literature. Haematologica 2006; 91(12 Suppl):ECR48.

35. Pilichowska ME, Fleming MD, Pinkus JL, et al. CD4+/CD56+ hematodermic neoplasm ("Blastic Natural Killer Cell Lymphoma") neoplastic cells express the immature dendritic cell marker BDCA-2 and produce interferon. Am J Clin Pathol 2007;128(3):445–53.

36. Hu SC-S, Tsai K-B, Chen G-S, et al. Infantile CD4+/CD56+ hematodermic neoplasm. Haematologica 2007;92(9):e91–3.

37. Hama A, Kudo K, Itzel BV, et al. Plasmacytoid dendritic cell leukemia in children. J Pediatr Hematol Oncol 2009;31(5):339–43.

38. Angelot-Delettre F, Roggy A, Frankel AE, et al. In vivo and in vitro sensitivity of blastic plasmacytoid dendritic cell neoplasm to SL-401, an interleukin-3 receptor targeted biologic agent. Haematologica 2015;100(2):223–30.

39. Alkharabsheh O, Frankel A. Clinical activity and tolerability of SL-401 (tagraxofusp): recombinant diphtheria toxin and interleukin-3 in hematologic malignancies. Biomedicines 2019;7(1):6.

40. Montero J, Stephansky J, Cai T, et al. Blastic plasmacytoid dendritic cell neoplasm is dependent on BCL2 and sensitive to venetoclax. Cancer Discov 2017;7(2):156–64.

41. DiNardo CD, Rausch CR, Benton C, et al. Clinical experience with the BCL 2-inhibitor venetoclax in combination therapy for relapsed and refractory acute myeloid leukemia and related myeloid malignancies. Am J Hematol 2018;93(3): 401–7.

42. Grushchak S, Joy C, Gray A, et al. Novel treatment of blastic plasmacytoid dendritic cell neoplasm: a case report. Medicine 2017;96(51):e9452.

43. Cai T, Galetto R, Gouble A, et al. Pre-clinical studies of anti-CD123 CAR-T cells for the treatment of blastic plasmacytoid dendritic cell neoplasm (BPDCN). Blood 2016;128(22):4039.

44. Menezes J, Acquadro F, Wiseman M, et al. Exome sequencing reveals novel and recurrent mutations with clinical impact in blastic plasmacytoid dendritic cell neoplasm. Leukemia 2014;28(4):823.

45. Laribi K, Denizon N, Ghnaya H, et al. Blastic plasmacytoid dendritic cell neoplasm: the first report of two cases treated by 5-Azacytidine. Eur J Haematol 2014;93(1):81–5.

46. Khwaja R, Daly A, Wong M, et al. Azacitidine in the treatment of blastic plasma-cytoid dendritic cell neoplasm: a report of 3 cases. Leuk Lymphoma 2016;57(11): 2720–2.
47. Pemmaraju N. Novel pathways and potential therapeutic strategies for blastic plasmacytoid dendritic cell neoplasm (BPDCN): CD123 and beyond. Curr Hematol Malig Rep 2017;12(6):510–2.
48. Emadali A, Hoghoughi N, Duley S, et al. Haploinsufficiency for NR3C1, the gene encoding the glucocorticoid receptor, in blastic plasmacytoid dendritic cell neoplasms. Blood 2016;127(24):3040–53.
49. Ceribelli M, Hou ZE, Kelly PN, et al. A druggable TCF4-and BRD4-dependent transcriptional network sustains malignancy in blastic plasmacytoid dendritic cell neoplasm. Cancer cell 2016;30(5):764–78.
50. Sakamoto K, Katayama R, Asaka R, et al. Recurrent 8q24 rearrangement in blastic plasmacytoid dendritic cell neoplasm: association with immunoblastoid cytomorphology, MYC expression, and drug response. Leukemia 2018;32(12): 2590–603.
51. Philippe L, Ceroi A, Bôle-Richard E, et al. Bortezomib as a new therapeutic approach for blastic plasmacytoid dendritic cell neoplasm. Haematologica 2017;102(11):1861–8.
52. Kharfan-Dabaja MA, Pemmaraju N, Mohty M. Therapeutic approaches for blastic plasmacytoid dendritic cell neoplasm: allogeneic hematopoietic cell transplantation and novel therapies. Clin Hematol Int 2019;1(1):2–9.
53. Deng W, Yang M, Kuang F, et al. Blastic plasmacytoid dendritic cell neoplasm in children: a review of two cases. Mol Clin Oncol 2017;7(4):709–15.
54. Berry DA, Zhou S, Higley H, et al. Association of minimal residual disease with clinical outcome in pediatric and adult acute lymphoblastic leukemia: a meta-analysis. JAMA Oncol 2017;3(7):e170580.

Blastic Plasmacytoid Dendritic Cell Neoplasm
The European Perspective

Eric Deconinck, MD, PhD

KEYWORDS

- BPDCN • Orphan disease • Network • International cooperation • Tagraxofusp
- Allogeneic transplantation • Europe

KEY POINTS

- The accurate diagnosis of BPDCN is the primary step for a better treatment of patients.
- The optimal care of BPDCN patients requires a national and probably an international collaboration.
- The social networks are probably a good option to inform patients and medical community on this rare disease.
- BPDCN could be a model for the development and the structuring of a concerted medical program for orphan tumors.

INTRODUCTION

Blastic plasmacytoid dendritic cell neoplasm (BPDCN) (ICD-O code 9727/3) has to be considered as an orphan tumoral disease.[1] The first description seems to have been reported in 1998 when Kameoka and colleagues[2] described a case as a cutaneous agranular CD2–/CD4+/CD56+ lymphoma. At the beginning of the twenty-first century, subsequent publications confirmed this emerging new entity. Now, since the 2008 edition of the World Health Organization Classification of Tumors of Hematopoietic and Lymphoid Tissues,[3] it is clearly identified and belongs to the acute myeloid leukemia-related precursor neoplasms; in 2016, BPDCN was even set out as a distinct entity in the scope myeloid neoplasms.[4] This attempt to better recognize the disease was conducted over the last few years and dealt with the biological spectrum of this new entity especially on the genetic and molecular level and was reported to numerous publications.[5–7] Despite this progress, and due to the rareness of the cases, an accurate diagnosis remains a real challenge for all the medical community and this is also the first step to an adapted treatment.[8,9] When the correct diagnosis is obtained, a tremendous challenge remains for the physician and the patient: What is

Hematology, CHU Besançon, Besançon Cedex 25030, France
E-mail addresses: edeconinck@chu-besancon.fr; eric.deconinck@univ-fcomte.fr
Twitter: @edocpatch (E.D.)

Hematol Oncol Clin N Am 34 (2020) 613–620
https://doi.org/10.1016/j.hoc.2020.01.012
0889-8588/20/© 2020 Elsevier Inc. All rights reserved.

hemonc.theclinics.com

the best treatment? Since 2018, no specific drug has demonstrated a clear and reproducible durable antitumoral effect until the approval of tragaxofusp (Elzonris, Stemline Therapeutics) in the United States.[10,11] Short retrospective series or collections of case reports have been published during the last decade, but no consensual therapeutic approach emerged.[8,9] In younger patients, acute leukemia-like regimens were described as providing high but short response rates and unfortunately the disease preferentially affected old patients.[12–15] The only largely recognized therapeutic approach is allogeneic hematopoietic cell transplantation, which represents the best consolidation strategy in fit eligible patients in remission, but this does not include the majority of patients who are more than 65 years old and with an altered clinical status and the presence of comorbidities.[14–19]

Considering all these characteristics, BPDCN is probably a good model of an orphan tumor with regard to the structuring and organization of a concerted medical program (diagnostic step, therapeutic step) on a nation-based or a transnational level, or even an international level. This is currently of special importance; the first dedicated treatment has been approved in the United States and has been submitted for near forthcoming approval to the European authorities.[10]

THE FRENCH EXPERIENCE

The first description of a "lymphoma," with the then unknown characteristics that could be attributed to a BPDCN localization, probably dates back to 1991 in a publication by Petrella and colleagues[20] French dermatologists and pathologists then occasionally reported case reports with similar biological features.[21–23] In the late 1990s and at the beginning of the twenty-first century several short series were reported in the literature, and 3 French groups, the Groupe d'Etude Immunologique des Leucémies curently named Cytométrie Hématologique Francophone (CytHem; https://www.cythem.fr), the Groupe Français de Cytogénétique Hématologique, and mainly the Groupe Francophone d'Hématologie Cellulaire (http://gfhc.fr/fr), as members of the French Society of Hematology (Société Française d'Hématologie [SFH], http://sfh.hematologie.net), started a collection of samples with these specific pathologic and immunologic features.[24,25] Petrella and colleagues[12,26] described a large series of 91 cases and reported the biological but also clinical characteristics of this newly defined entity in detail. In 2008, Garnache-Ottou and colleagues[27] proposed an immunologic score to extend the diagnostic pattern of BPDCN based on part on this large collection. Since 2004, all new French cases matching the defined criteria were systematically referenced, and the data have contributed to the creation of the French BPDCN Network (**Fig. 1**).[28] This collaboration between all French centers, by permitting a centralized review in a dedicated laboratory, allows to ensure an accurate diagnosis of all new cases of BPDCN that could be specifically counted and identified; several publications have emerged from this collaborative work.[28,29] After this first diagnostic step, the question of an adapted treatment rises. Our preliminary question was to collect the treatments generally used in patients with BPDCN and to identify the therapeutic approaches in France for the usual care of this disease. Based on the French BPDCN Network collection, the author identified the treatments received by each patient in a series of 89 well-documented cases.[14,15] In brief, a quarter of them was treated with a palliative intent and the patients received supportive care only or oral chemotherapy with steroids; another quarter was treated like acute leukemia patients with acute myeloid or lymphoid leukemia chemotherapy regimens; the third quarter received lymphoma regimens, such as CHOP; and the last quarter a more original regimen based on methotrexate and asparaginase.[30–32] According to

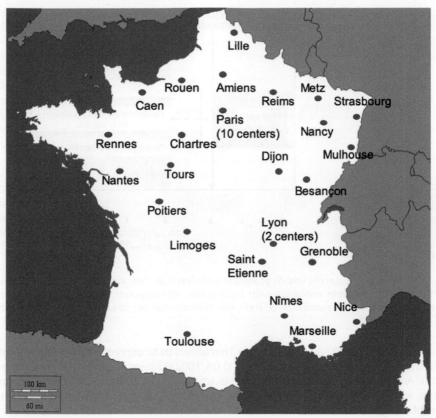

Fig. 1. French centers in the blastic plasmacytoid dendritic cell neoplasm network. (*Courtesy of* Francine Garnache-Ottou, Besançon, France.)

our results presented at the 57th American Society of Hematology meeting in 2015, and recently updated, acute leukemia regimens offer a higher complete remission rate and clearly the best overall survival if an allogeneic hematopoietic transplantation could be offered to responding patients. The results are similar with the methotrexate-asparaginase-based regimen but are significantly inferior in terms of response rate and survival with the CHOP regimen. These data also confirm the crucial role of allogeneic hematopoietic stem cell transplantation (HCT) with an overall survival of 40% with a long follow-up in transplanted patients. These data are similar to and confirm those already published.[12,26] Currently there is no consensus concerning the first-line treatment of BPDCN patients.[33] The author decided in 2016 to conduct a phase II trial, granted by the French National Institute of Cancer (Inca, PHRC-K16-093), to prospectively evaluate the real interest of the methotrexate-asparaginase regimen in combination with idarubicine (**Fig. 2**). The author has previously demonstrated in a preclinical model that this drug is one of the most effective in the eradication of BPDCN cells in in vitro and animal models.[28] This trial is open for inclusions since January 2019 (ClinicalTrials.gov identifier: NCT03599960) and recruited 5 patients in the last 6 months. During this same period, the author identified 5 patients who were noneligible due to older age or unsuitable clinical conditions with an altered clinical status and comorbidities (personal unpublished data). This trial also offers the opportunity to exhaustively identify new BPDCN patients in France and to centralize all

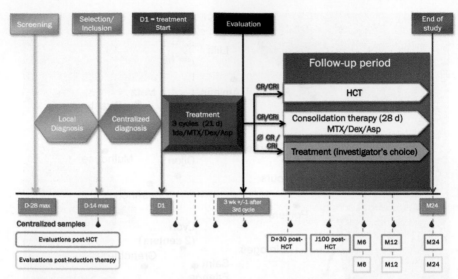

Fig. 2. Scheme of the current French prospective clinical trial. Asp, asparaginase; CR, complete remission; CRi, complete remission with incomplete hematopoietic recovery; D, day; Dex, dexamethasone; HCT, hematopoietic stem cell transplantation; Ida, idarubicin; M, month; MTX, methotrexate.

diagnostics with 1 to 2 new patients/mo. This allows us to confirm the real incidence of BPDCN in France with a ratio of 0.03 to 0.04/100,000 people (personal unpublished data). Another prospective trial (phase I) is also ongoing in France for relapsing patients with the use of an anti-CD123 chemo-conjugated monoclonal antibody as part of a larger international trial (ClinicalTrials.gov identifier: NCT03386513).

In 2019 in France, the diagnosis process for BPDCN is clearly established with a unique central laboratory that collects all cases and can confirm, register, and explore the biological features. This evolutive collection serves for genomic and cytogenetic forthcoming studies. For the first time, 2 prospective clinical trials are ongoing and have allowed the constitution of a central platform and a network of physicians to optimize the medical care and provide access to the best treatments for all BPDCN patients in the era of emerging anti-CD123 targeted therapy, for example, or new drug combinations.[34,35]

THE EUROPEAN PERSPECTIVE

At this time there is no real structure concerning BPDCN care among the different European countries. The European Group for Blood and Marrow Transplantation (EBMT) centralized data concerning all transplanted patients in Europe and a series was reported in 2013 focusing on allogeneic HCT and collecting data from Austria, France, Germany, Italy, Spain, and the United Kingdom.[17] Published data from other countries are scarce especially in Eastern Europe; case reports have been identified in Turkey[36,37] and a short series from Poland has been published.[38] Several Italian[8,39,40] and Spanish[41,42] teams have reported significant experience with the diagnosis and the treatment of BPDCN, but there was no clear national structure. In Greece, the Hellenic Dendritic Cell Leukemia Study Group identified a cohort of 22 patients.[43] Currently in European countries, BPDCN is generally considered as a specific form of acute leukemia and included in the leukemia working program of each country, especially with regard to treatment; eligible patients are offered an allogeneic HCT, which remains the best consolidation treatment. With the arrival of targeted therapy focusing the CD123 pathway, BPDCN will become an appropriate disease for the development of these molecules.[34,35] Because of the difficulties in diagnostic procedures and the rarity of the disease it is important that European countries collaborate to build a real European network. We can take advantage of the existence of 2 well-structured and efficient hematological societies, EBMT and the European Hematology Association, to initiate this work. There are also probably some opportunities by using the preexisting networks on rare diseases, such as Orphanet (www.orpha.net), a 37-country network, cofunded by the European Commission, or EURORDIS-Rare Diseases Europe (www.eurordis.org), which is a unique, nonprofit alliance of rare disease patient organizations even if those predominantly deal with inherited disorders rather than with rare tumors. An interesting and contemporary experience is the use of social networks as described and successfully used by Pemmaraju and colleagues[44–46] in the United States: "The use of social media, and in particular, Twitter, for professional use among healthcare providers is rapidly increasing across the world. One medical subspecialty that is, leading the integration of this new platform for communication into daily practice and for information dissemination to the general public is the field of hematology/oncology." This is especially true with the introduction on Twitter of the hashtag #BPDCN and the @BPDCNInfo count, which allow a large and rapid diffusion of information into the medical community but also within a large population, including the concerned patients: "Twitter has served as a platform for academic discussion, a method for knowledge dissemination directly from medical meetings, and a venue for patient caregiver and support groups."[45,46] In a recent analysis of Tweet metrics (9/2018). Pemmaraju and colleagues[46] identified almost 300 followers and 1000 tweets, including #BPDCN with a majority of retweets. This phenomenon is emerging and is much less frequent than for other diseases, but it is probably one of the future paths to ensure that the current knowledge and the best access to adequate medical care is available for these patients with a rare disease.

SUMMARY

BPDCN is now well defined but remains a real orphan tumor; accurate diagnosis is still difficult to establish. The first dedicated and targeted treatment will become available soon in Europe and several new therapeutic approaches are emerging. Collaboration is the key for diagnosis and treatment of this rare disease, and we all have to work together: the medical community and the patients throughout European countries, with the help of EBMT and EHA, via social networks to ensure the best and equitable medical care to all BPDCN patients.

DISCLOSURE

E. Deconinck belongs to the EBMT and SFH, is a member of a subcommittee of the Agence française de la Biomédecine, and participates in boards for Stemline therapeutics and ImunoGen.

REFERENCES

1. Swerdlow SH, Campo E, Harris NL, et al, editors. WHO classification of tumours of haematopoietic and lymphoid tissues. World Health Organization classification of tumours, vol. 2, 4th edition. Lyon (France): International Agency for Research on Cancer; 2017.

2. Kameoka J, Ichinohasama R, Tanaka M, et al. A cutaneous agranular CD2–CD4+ CD56+ "lymphoma": report of two cases and review of the literature. Am J Clin Pathol 1998;110(4):478–88.

3. Vardiman JW, Thiele J, Arber DA, et al. The 2008 revision of the World Health Organization (WHO) classification of myeloid neoplasms and acute leukemia: rationale and important changes. Blood 2009;114:937–51.

4. Arber DA, Orazi A, Hasserjian R, et al. The 2016 revision to the World Health Organization classification of myeloid neoplasms and acute leukemia. Blood 2016; 127(20):2391–405.

5. Kubota S, Tokunaga K, Umezu T, et al. Lineage-specific RUNX2 super-enhancer activates MYC and promotes the development of blastic plasmacytoid dendritic cell neoplasm. Nat Commun 2019;10(1):1653.

6. Hamadeh F, Awadallah A, Meyerson HJ, et al. Flow cytometry identifies a spectrum of maturation in myeloid neoplasms having plasmacytoid dendritic cell differentiation. Cytometry B Clin Cytom 2019;98(1):43–51.

7. Sapienza MR, Abate F, Melle F, et al. Blastic plasmacytoid dendritic cell neoplasm: genomics mark epigenetic dysregulation as a primary therapeutic target. Haematologica 2019;104(4):729–37.

8. Sapienza MR, Pileri A, Derenzini E, et al. Blastic plasmacytoid dendritic cell neoplasm: state of the art and prospects. Cancers (Basel) 2019;11(5) [pii:E595].

9. Venugopal S, Zhou S, El Jamal SM, et al. Blastic plasmacytoid dendritic cell neoplasm—current insights. Clin Lymphoma Myeloma Leuk 2019;19(9):545–54.

10. Economides MP, McCue D, Lane AA, et al. Tagraxofusp, the first CD123-targeted therapy and first targeted treatment for blastic plasmacytoid dendritic cell neoplasm. Expert Rev Clin Pharmacol 2019;12(10):941–6.

11. Pemmaraju N, Lane AA, Sweet KL, et al. Tagraxofusp in blastic plasmacytoid dendritic-cell neoplasm. N Engl J Med 2019;380(17):1628–37.

12. Julia F, Petrella T, Beylot-Barry M, et al. Blastic plasmacytoid dendritic cell neoplasm: clinical features in 90 patients. Br J Dermatol 2013;169(3):579–86.

13. Taylor J, Haddadin M, Upadhyay VA, et al. Multicenter analysis of outcomes in blastic plasmacytoid dendritic cell neoplasm offers a pretargeted therapy benchmark. Blood 2019;134(8):678–87.

14. Poret E, Vidal C, Desbrosses Y, et al. How to treat blastic plasmacytoid dendritic cell neoplasm (BPDCN) patients: results on 86 patients of the French BPDCN network. Blood 2015;126(23):456.

15. Garnache-Ottou F, Vidal C, Biichlé S, et al. How should we diagnose and treat blastic plasmacytoid dendritic cell neoplasm (BPDCN) patients? Blood Advances 2019;3(24):4238-4251.

16. Dietrich S, Andrulis M, Hegenbart U, et al. Blastic plasmacytoid dendritic cell neoplasia (BPDC) in elderly patients: results of a treatment algorithm employing allogeneic stem cell transplantation with moderately reduced conditioning intensity. Biol Blood Marrow Transplant 2011;17(8):1250–4.

17. Roos-Weil D, Dietrich S, Boumendil A, et al, European Group for Blood and Marrow Transplantation Lymphoma, Pediatric Diseases, and Acute Leukemia Working Parties. Stem cell transplantation can provide durable disease control in blastic plasmacytoid dendritic cell neoplasm: a retrospective study from the European Group for Blood and Marrow Transplantation. Blood 2013;121(3): 440–6.

18. Kharfan-Dabaja MA, Al Malki MM, Deotare U, et al. Haematopoietic cell transplantation for blastic plasmacytoid dendritic cell neoplasm: a North American multicentre collaborative study. Br J Haematol 2017;179(5):781–9.

19. Kharfan-Dabaja MA, Reljic T, Murthy HS, et al. Allogeneic hematopoietic cell transplantation is an effective treatment for blastic plasmacytoid dendritic cell neoplasm in first complete remission: systematic review and meta-analysis. Clin Lymphoma Myeloma Leuk 2018;18(11):703–9.
20. Petrella T, Bron A, Foulet A, et al. Report of a primary lymphoma of the conjunctiva. A lymphoma of MALT origin? Pathol Res Pract 1991;187(1):78–84.
21. Vitte F, Fabiani B, Bénet C, et al. Specific skin lesions in chronic myelomonocytic leukemia: a spectrum of myelomonocytic and dendritic cell proliferations: a study of 42 cases. Am J Surg Pathol 2012;36(9):1302–16.
22. Dalle S, Beylot-Barry M, Bagot M, et al. Blastic plasmacytoid dendritic cell neoplasm: is transplantation the treatment of choice? Br J Dermatol 2010; 162(1):74–9.
23. Petrella T, Facchetti F. Tumoral aspects of plasmacytoid dendritic cells: what do we know in 2009? Autoimmunity 2010;43(3):210–4.
24. Béné MC, Feuillard J, Jacob MC, Groupe d'Etude Immunologique des Leucémies. Plasmacytoid dendritic cells: from the plasmacytoid T-cell to type 2 dendritic cells CD4+CD56+ malignancies. Semin Hematol 2003;40(3):257–66.
25. Leroux D, Mugneret F, Callanan M, et al. CD4(+), CD56(+) DC2 acute leukemia is characterized by recurrent clonal chromosomal changes affecting 6 major targets: a study of 21 cases by the Groupe Français de Cytogénétique Hématologique. Blood 2002;99(11):4154–9.
26. Julia F, Dalle S, Duru G, et al. Blastic plasmacytoid dendritic cell neoplasms: clinico-immunohistochemical correlations in a series of 91 patients. Am J Surg Pathol 2014;38(5):673–80.
27. Garnache-Ottou F, Feuillard J, Ferrand C, et al, GOELAMS, GEIL study. Extended diagnostic criteria for plasmacytoid dendritic cell leukaemia. Br J Haematol 2009; 145(5):624–36.
28. Angelot-Delettre F, Roggy A, Frankel AE, et al. In vivo and in vitro sensitivity of blastic plasmacytoid dendritic cell neoplasm to SL-401, an interleukin-3 receptor targeted biologic agent. Haematologica 2015;100(2):223–30.
29. Emadali A, Hoghoughi N, Duley S, et al. Haploinsufficiency for NR3C1, the gene encoding the glucocorticoid receptor, in blastic plasmacytoid dendritic cell neoplasms. Blood 2016;127(24):3040–53.
30. Gilis L, Lebras L, Bouafia-Sauvy F, et al. Sequential combination of high dose methotrexate and L-asparaginase followed by allogeneic transplant: a first-line strategy for CD4+/CD56+ hematodermic neoplasm. Leuk Lymphoma 2012; 53(8):1633–7.
31. Fontaine J, Thomas L, Balme B, et al. Haematodermic CD4+CD56+ neoplasm: complete remission after methotrexate-asparaginase treatment. Clin Exp Dermatol 2009;34(5):e43–5.
32. Gruson B, Vaida I, Merlusca L, et al. L-Asparaginase with methotrexate and dexamethasone is an effective treatment combination in blastic plasmacytoid dendritic cell neoplasm. Br J Haematol 2013;163(4):543–5.
33. Laribi K, Denizon N, Besançon A, et al. Blastic plasmacytoid dendritic cell neoplasm: from origin of the cell to targeted therapies. Biol Blood Marrow Transplant 2016;22(8):1357–67.
34. Testa U, Pelosi E, Castelli G. CD123 as a therapeutic target in the treatment of hematological malignancies. Cancers (Basel) 2019;11(9) [pii:E1358].
35. Marmouset V, Joris M, Merlusca L, et al. The lenalidomide/bortezomib/dexamethasone regimen for the treatment of blastic plasmacytoid dendritic cell neoplasm. Hematol Oncol 2019;37(4):487–9.

36. Dhariwal S, Gupta M. A case of blastic plasmacytoid dendritic cell neoplasm with unusual presentation. [[Sıradışı Başlangıçlı Bir Blastik Plazmasitoid Dendritik Hücreli Neoplazi Olgusu]]. Turk J Haematol 2019;36(1):55–6.
37. Hale B, Özsan N, Hekimgil M, et al. Report on three patients with blastic plasmacytoid dendritic cell neoplasm. [[Blastik Plazmasitoid Dentritik Hücreli Neoplazmlı Üç Olgu Sunumu]]. Turk J Haematol 2018;35(3):211–2.
38. Owczarczyk-Saczonek A, Sokołowska-Wojdyło M, Olszewska B, et al. Clinicopathologic retrospective analysis of blastic plasmacytoid dendritic cell neoplasms. Postepy Dermatol Alergol 2018;35(2):128–38.
39. Pileri A, Delfino C, Grandi V, et al. Blastic plasmacytoid dendritic cell neoplasm (BPDCN): the cutaneous sanctuary. G Ital Dermatol Venereol 2012;147(6):603–8.
40. Pagano L, Valentini CG, Grammatico S, et al. Blastic plasmacytoid dendritic cell neoplasm: diagnostic criteria and therapeutical approaches. Br J Haematol 2016; 174(2):188–202.
41. Martín-Martín L, Almeida J, Pomares H, et al. Blastic plasmacytoid dendritic cell neoplasm frequently shows occult central nervous system involvement at diagnosis and benefits from intrathecal therapy. Oncotarget 2016;7(9):10174–81.
42. Martín-Martín L, López A, Vidriales B, et al. Classification and clinical behavior of blastic plasmacytoid dendritic cell neoplasms according to their maturation-associated immunophenotypic profile. Oncotarget 2015;6(22):19204–16.
43. Tsagarakis Nj, Kentrou Na, Papadimitriou Ka, et al. Acute lymphoplasmacytoid dendritic cell (DC2) leukemia: results from the hellenic dendritic cell leukemia study group. Leuk Res 2010;34:438–46.
44. Pemmaraju N, Utengen A, Gupta V, et al. Blastic plasmacytoid dendritic cell neoplasm (BPDCN) on social media: #BPDCN-increasing exposure over two years since inception of a disease-specific twitter community. Curr Hematol Malig Rep 2018;13(6):581–7.
45. Pemmaraju N, Utengen A, Gupta V, et al. Analysis of first-year twitter metrics of a rare disease community for blastic plasmacytoid dendritic cell neoplasm (BPDCN) on social media: #BPDCN. Curr Hematol Malig Rep 2017;12(6):592–7.
46. Pemmaraju N, Gupta V, Thompson MA, et al. Social media and internet resources for patients with blastic plasmacytoid dendritic cell neoplasm (BPDCN). Curr Hematol Malig Rep 2016;11(6):462–7.

Hematopoietic Cell Transplant for Blastic Plasmacytoid Dendritic Cell Neoplasm

Mohamed A. Kharfan-Dabaja, MD, MBA[a],*,
Mohamad Cherry, MD[b]

KEYWORDS

- Allogeneic hematopoietic cell transplant • Autologous hematopoietic cell transplant
- Blastic plasmacytoid dendritic cell neoplasm • Survival

KEY POINTS

- Blastic plasmacytoid dendritic cell neoplasm (BPDCN) is a rare aggressive hematologic malignancy derived from precursors of plasmacytoid dendritic cells. Historically, BPDCN has had few available treatment options and a poor prognosis.
- The emergence of novel targeted therapies, namely tagraxofusp, has changed the treatment landscape of BPDCN, but data are lacking regarding the long-term durability of responses.
- Allogeneic hematopoietic cell transplant is the recommended front-line consolidative treatment modality for patients with BPDCN who achieve first complete remission and are fit for the procedure.
- As new therapies that are better tolerated continue to emerge, it will be important to evaluate the role of postallograft maintenance/consolidation in order to reduce the risk of BPDCN relapse.
- In addition, advances in immune oncology and T-cell engineering have brought novel cellular therapies that are improving the prognosis of several hematologic malignancies, namely chimeric antigen receptor T-cell therapy.

INTRODUCTION

Blastic plasmacytoid dendritic cell neoplasm (BPDCN) is generally a clinically aggressive hematologic malignancy derived from precursors of plasmacytoid dendritic

---

Funding: No funding for this work.
[a] Division of Hematology-Oncology, Blood and Marrow Transplantation Program, Mayo Clinic, 4500 San Pablo Road, Mangurian Building 3rd Floor, Jacksonville, FL 32224, USA; [b] Morristown Medical Center, Atlantic Hematology Oncology, 100 Madison Avenue, Morristown, NJ 07960, USA
* Corresponding author.
E-mail address: KharfanDabaja.Mohamed@Mayo.Edu

Hematol Oncol Clin N Am 34 (2020) 621–629
https://doi.org/10.1016/j.hoc.2020.01.009
0889-8588/20/© 2020 Elsevier Inc. All rights reserved.

hemonc.theclinics.com

cells.[1-3] Historically, BPDCN has had few available treatment options and a poor prognosis. Treatment was limited to combination chemotherapy regimens used to treat acute leukemias, lymphoblastic or myeloid in origin, and aggressive lymphomas.[2,4] However, these treatments were not curative in BPDCN, and anticipated median overall survival (OS) ranged from 8 to 14 months at best.[4,5] Besides, toxicities associated with these regimens limited the ability to prescribe them to patients of more advanced age, who represent a significant proportion of patients with BPDCN, or to those with associated comorbidities.

Emergence of novel targeted therapies, namely tagraxofusp, has changed the treatment landscape of BPDCN.[6] A recently published, open-label, multicenter cohort of 47 patients (first line = 32, previously treated = 15) showed encouraging results in this disease.[6] The primary outcome was to assess the combined rate of complete response (CR) and clinical CR in treatment-naive patients.[6] Treatment with tagraxofusp resulted in an overall response rate (ORR) of 90% and the primary study outcome was met in 72%.[6] The 2-year OS was 52%, which represents a significant improvement vis à vis outcomes with conventional therapies.[6] Published literature in BPDCN shows that patients with relapsed or refractory disease have a poor prognosis when treated with conventional chemotherapy or even with hematopoietic cell transplant (HCT).[2,4,5,7] In this regard, tagraxofusp also showed a lower efficacy in patients with BPDCN who had failed prior therapies, with a reported ORR of 67% and a short median OS of only 8.5 months.[6] The most common adverse events associated with tagraxofusp were transaminitis ($\geq$60%), hypoalbuminemia (55%), peripheral edema (51%), and thrombocytopenia (49%).[6] One particularly serious adverse event, namely capillary leak syndrome, was described in 19% and was associated with 1 death in each of the dose subgroups.[6] Although responses to tagraxofusp are encouraging, data are lacking regarding the long-term durability of responses. In the study by Pemmaraju and colleagues,[6] 10 (34%) of 29 patients who received tagraxofusp in the front-line setting ended up receiving an allogeneic HCT (allo-HCT) as further consolidation.

Despite the absence of randomized data comparing chemotherapy versus allo-HCT, the latter has become the de facto option for patients with BPDCN who achieve a first complete remission (CR1) and, at the same time, are deemed fit for the procedure.[7] Data supporting the role of allo-HCT are limited to multicenter observational studies or registry data.[8-11]

This article provides a comprehensive assessment of the role of HCT in patients with BPDCN. It also reviews the emergence of novel T cell–based cellular treatments, namely chimeric antigen receptor T-cell (CART) therapy.

HEMATOPOIETIC CELL TRANSPLANT FOR BLASTIC PLASMACYTOID DENDRITIC CELL NEOPLASM

The predominance of published data on allo-HCT suggests an inherent bias that favors offering allo-HCT (rather than autologous HCT [auto-HCT]) for patients with BPDCN. The published literature on HCT, allogeneic or autologous, for BPDCN is summarized here.

Allogeneic Hematopoietic Cell Transplant

Allo-HCT is a potentially curative therapy for various hematologic malignancies and benign blood disorders.[12,13] Several studies have shown that donor effector cells, namely T lymphocytes, play an important role in disease eradication in myeloid and lymphoid malignancies treated with an allo-HCT.[14-16]

To our knowledge, there has never been a randomized controlled trial that compared allo-HCT with conventional chemotherapy or novel therapies in patients with BPDCN. However, offering an allo-HCT has become the standard treatment approach for fit patients with BPDCN who achieve CR1. Published data show that the efficacy of allo-HCT is less encouraging in patients offered the procedure at a later stage of the disease. Before 2012, most of the published data assessing the role of allo-HCT in BPDCN were limited to a small case series of fewer than 10 patients.[7,17]

Roos-Weil and colleagues[8] published an analysis from the European Society for Blood and Marrow Transplantation (EBMT) registry reporting postallograft outcomes in patients with BPDCN. The investigators had originally identified 139 patients, but, after central review of immunophenotype and pathology reports, the diagnosis of BPDCN was confirmed in only 39 patients.[8] Thirty-four patients, median age of 41 years, received an allo-HCT for BPDCN, following a myeloablative conditioning (MAC; n = 25) or reduced-intensity conditioning (RIC; n = 9) regimen.[8] A total of 19 patients (MAC = 15, RIC = 4) were in CR1 at the time of allo-HCT, representing 56% of the allografted population.[8] The cell source was mostly (n = 19, 56%) bone marrow (BM) and most donors were unrelated (n = 23, 68%).[8] The investigators reported that 16 (47%) allograft recipients were alive at a median follow-up of 28 months.[8] The 3-year cumulative incidences of relapse, disease-free survival (DFS), and OS were 32%, 33%, and 41% respectively.[8] The investigators showed that patients who received the allo-HCT in CR1 had almost 2-fold better OS compared with those allografted in a more advanced stage (52% vs 29%, $P = .06$).[8] The small number of RIC allo-HCT recipients (n = 9) was a limiting factor in evaluating the impact of regimen intensity (ie, MAC vs RIC allo-HCT) in postallograft outcomes.[8]

A smaller registry study from the Japanese Society for Hematopoietic Cell Transplantation described post–allo-HCT outcomes in 14 patients (male = 11, 79%) with BPDCN with a median age of 58 years.[9] Most of the patients (n = 12, 86%) had skin involvement at initial presentation, which is characteristic of this disease.[9] Ten (71%) of 14 cases were in CR1 at the time of allo-HCT and the remainder were allografted in CR2 (n = 2, 14%) or refractory disease (n = 2, 14%).[9] BM was the most commonly used cell source (n = 8, 57%).[9] MAC regimens were most commonly prescribed (n = 8, 57%).[9] The investigators reported an encouraging 4-year progression-free survival (PFS) and OS of 60% and 69%, respectively, for patients allografted in CR1.[9] These results are impressive when considering that the median age of allografted patients was 58 years.[9]

A multicenter observational study from North America evaluated the efficacy of allo-HCT in 37 patients with BPDCN.[10] The median age of allografted patients was 50 years and most were male (n = 29, 78%).[10] Most patients had skin and marrow involvement at initial presentation.[10] In total, 20 (54%) patients received an MAC regimen using peripheral blood stem cells (n = 25, 68%).[10] Most patients were prescribed the allo-HCT in CR1 (n = 28, 76%).[10] The investigators reported a 1-year cumulative incidence of nonrelapse mortality of 25%, and 3-year OS and PFS of 58% and 55%, respectively, for all allo-HCT recipients.[10] Consistent with other studies, the 3-year OS and PFS for those allografted in CR1 was better at 74% and 69%, respectively. Multivariate analysis suggests that patients in CR1 benefit the most from the allo-HCT.[10] This study did not find an advantage in OS with more intensive MAC regimens (hazard ratio = 1.01; 95% confidence interval = 0.13–7.90), with the limitation of a small sample size.[10]

A study from several French transplant centers involving 43 patients (male = 29, 67%), median age of 57 years, who received an allo-HCT for BPDCN using an MAC (n = 14, 33%) or RIC/nonmyeloablative (NMA) (n = 29, 67%) conditioning regimen reported a 2-year OS of 52%.[11] The investigators did not report a difference in 2-year OS in relation to the intensity of the conditioning regimen (RIC/NMA = 50% vs MAC = 57%, P = .91).[11] Although there was a 5-fold higher 2-year cumulative incidence of relapse with RIC/NMA regimens (7% vs 36%), this difference was not statistically significant (P = .137).[11] The lack of benefit with MAC regimens can be explained in part by the small sample size and by the fact that most cases receiving RIC/NMA (79%) or MAC regimens (86%) were in CR1 at the time of allografting.[11]

A recently published systematic review/meta-analysis involving 128 patients with BPDCN showed pooled OS of 67% for patients allografted in CR1 versus 7% for patients who received an allo-HCT beyond CR1.[18] These findings further highlight the importance of offering the procedure in CR1. The pooled OS based on intensity of the conditioning regimen shows 55% for MAC and 44% for RIC regimens.[18] These studies are summarized in **Table 1**.

Autologous Hematopoietic Cell Transplant

Data assessing the role of auto-HCT in BPDCN are limited to single case reports or smaller studies.[7,9,10] The Japanese study using registry data also included 11 patients with BPDCN, median age of 57 years, treated with an auto-HCT between 2003 and 2013.[9] All 11 patients were in CR1 at the time of auto-HCT, and the median time from diagnosis to autografting was 6 months.[9] The reported 4-year OS was 82%.[9] Other observational studies have shown less encouraging outcomes when using auto-HCT for BPDCN. Reimer and colleagues[19] reported 4 patients with BPDCN who received an auto-HCT in CR1 (n = 3) or in partial response (n = 1). Three of the 4 cases eventually died of relapse, within less than 2 years from autografting.[19] In addition, the aforementioned multicenter North American observational study of 8 patients, median age of 67 years, treated with an auto-HCT in CR1 (n = 5), or greater than or equal to CR2 (n = 2), or with primary induction failure (n = 1) showed a dismal 1-year OS of 11%.[10] One registry study from EBMT listed 5 patients with BPDCN who received an auto-HCT as part of their treatment.[8] However, the investigators did not report any data for this subgroup.[8] Differences between the Japanese[9] and the North American[10] studies include a younger population (median age 57 vs 67 years) and a higher percentage of CR1 cases (100% vs 63%) in the former. The small number of cases limits the ability to recommend an auto-HCT as a standard approach to patients with BPDCN.

Other T Cell–Based Cellular Therapies

Advances in immune oncology and T-cell engineering have brought novel cellular therapies that are improving the prognosis of several hematologic malignancies.[20–22] One major prerequisite for success is identifying actionable targets that affect key survival mechanisms. Cluster of differentiation (CD) 19 has proved to be such a target for large B-cell lymphomas, with one of the commercially approved anti-CD19 CART products, axicabtagene ciloleucel, showing encouraging 2-year OS of 50% in the relapsed/refractory setting.[20]

In the case of BPDCN, CD123 represents an attractive target for T cell–based immunotherapy.[23,24] Mardiros and colleagues[25] described promising preclinical data using lentiviral vectors encoding CD123-targeting CARTs against tumor cell lines and primary acute myeloid leukemia (AML) samples expressing CD123. The investigators confirmed in vivo antileukemic activity of CD123 CARTs in a xenogeneic model of systemic AML showing better survival for mice treated with CD123 CARTs.[25] Guzman and colleagues[26] developed an allogeneic CART platform using T cells from third-party healthy donors to generate engineered T cells targeting CD123 (UCART123). To reduce the potential for engineered T cells to cause graft-versus-host disease,

Table 1
Allogeneic hematopoietic cell transplant in blastic plasmacytoid dendritic cell neoplasm

Study	Study Type	Number of Patients	Median Age, Range (y)	CR1 at Time of Allo-HCT	MAC vs RIC Conditioning	Survival Outcomes (All Patients)	Survival Outcomes (CR1 Patients)
Roos-Weil et al,[8] 2013	EBMT registry	34	41 (10–70)	56%	MAC = 74% RIC = 26%	DFS = 33% OS = 41% (3 y)	DFS = 36% OS = 52% (3 y)
Aoki et al,[9] 2015	Japanese registry	14	58 (17–64)	71%	MAC = 57% RIC = 43%	—	PFS = 60% OS = 69% (4 y)
Kharfan-Dabaja et al,[10] 2017	Multicenter, observational, North America	37	50 (14–74)	76%	MAC = 54% RIC = 46%	PFS = 55% OS = 58% (3-y)	PFS = 69% OS = 74% (3-y)
Leclerc et al,[11] 2017	Multicenter, observational, France	43	57 (20–72)	79%	MAC = 33% RIC = 67%	DFS = 45% OS = 52% (2-y)	—
Kharfan-Dabaja et al,[18] 2018	Systematic review/meta-analysis	128	—	-	MAC = 4 studies (67 patients) RIC = 4 studies (61 patients)	Pooled DFS/PFS = 44% OS = 50% From 4 studies (128 patients)	Pooled DFS/PFS = 53% OS = 67% From 3 studies (57 patients)

investigators disrupted the TCRα gene using gene editing technology and subsequently eliminated TCRα/β-positive cells.[26] In vitro, UCART123 eliminated AML cells and had minimum effect on normal cells,[26] and in a xenograft model UCART123 treatment also eliminated the leukemic cells and improved OS.[26] Two clinical trials evaluating UCART123 are currently accruing patients (data from ClinicalTrials.gov accessed September 29, 2019). One study represents a phase 1 open-label dose escalation study (ClinicalTrials.gov identifier: NCT04106076) in patients with newly diagnosed CD123-positive adverse genetic risk AML as defined by the 2017 European LeukemiaNet classification.[27] The second is also a phase 1 dose-finding study in relapsed, refractory, or newly diagnosed patients with AML with poor prognosis (ClinicalTrials.gov identifier: NCT03190278). Other clinical trials evaluating the safety and efficacy of autologous anti-CD123 CARTs are also underway throughout the world.

Al-Hussaini and colleagues[28] reported promising preclinical work using a dual-affinity retargeting (DART) molecule generated from antibodies against CD3 and CD123, designed to redirect T cells against CD123-expressing AML blasts. The CD33xCD123 DART binds to both human CD3 and CD123 to mediate T-cell activation and proliferation, among others.[28]

DISCUSSION

Allo-HCT is currently the recommended front-line consolidative treatment modality for patients with BPDCN who achieve CR1 and are fit for the procedure. Given the superior OS observed in allo-HCT in CR1,[18] patients with BPDCN should be promptly referred to transplant centers to initiate the process of searching for a suitable human leukocyte antigen–compatible donor, confirming eligibility for the procedure, and proceeding with allo-HCT in a timely manner. For patients who are referred for allo-HCT at a later stage of the disease, outcomes are less encouraging, and offering the procedure should be considered on a case-by-case basis and/or in the context of a clinical trial, if available. To our knowledge, there are no strong data supporting use of MAC versus RIC allo-HCT regimens in patients with BPDCN. Intuitively, younger patients who are fit for the procedure are more likely to be prescribed intensive MAC regimens, whereas RIC allo-HCT would be preferentially offered to older patients who are perceived to be less fit to tolerate intensive doses of chemotherapy or chemoimmunotherapy.

It is possible that with the emergence of novel therapies such as tagraxofusp, which has been shown to be relatively well tolerated even in older patients (median age of 70 years), allo-HCT would potentially be offered to patients who were precluded in the past because of their inability to receive intensive induction chemotherapy regimens used for acute leukemias.[6] Note that 34% of patients treated with tagraxofusp in the front-line setting ended up eventually receiving an allo-HCT.[6]

Pertaining to auto-HCT, data are scanty and show conflicting results regarding the efficacy of this treatment modality. Although the aforementioned Japanese study showed a 4-year OS exceeding 80%, there were only 11 young patients, median age of 57 years, who were treated with an autograft in CR1.[9] By contrast, the North American, multicenter, observational study showed a poor 1-year OS of 11% when the procedure was offered to 8 older patients, median age of 67 years, with only 5 patients (63%) in CR1 at the time of the procedure.[10] These findings limit the ability to recommend auto-HCT as a standard option in BPDCN. More studies are needed to better understand the role of auto-HCT for BPDCN, in our opinion.

T cell–engineered therapies, namely CART, are revolutionizing the treatment of CD19-expressing lymphoid malignancies. For myeloid malignancies, identifying key actionable targets that do not result in prohibitive myelotoxicity is of paramount importance. Preclinical data targeting CD123 are promising and studies evaluating the safety and efficacy of anti-CD123 CARTs are currently ongoing.

There are several remaining challenges that need to be addressed in order to continue to improve the outcomes of BPDCN. One major challenge is accurately diagnosing these patients early in the disease course. This challenge is shown by the fact that only 39 of the 139 originally identified cased in the EBMT study were later confirmed as BPDCN.[8] Accordingly, all cases with a presumed AML diagnosis who have skin involvement need to be thoroughly evaluated by an experienced hematopathologist to confirm or rule out the diagnosis of BPDCN. Moreover, as new therapies that are better tolerated continue to emerge, it will be important to evaluate the role of postallograft maintenance/consolidation in order to reduce the risk of BPDCN relapse.[6,29,30] It will ultimately require a large collaborative research effort from transplant centers, considering the relatively low incidence of BPDCN.

CONFLICT OF INTEREST (PAST 24 MONTHS)

M.A. Kharfan-Dabaja: consultancy for Daiichi Sankyo and Pharmacyclics. M. Cherry: consultancy for Celgene, Incyte, and Abbvie.

REFERENCES

1. Chaperot L, Bendriss N, Manches O, et al. Identification of a leukemic counterpart of the plasmacytoid dendritic cells. Blood 2001;97(10):3210–7.
2. Feuillard J, Jacob MC, Valensi F, et al. Clinical and biologic features of CD4(+) CD56(+) malignancies. Blood 2002;99(5):1556–63.
3. Petrella T, Comeau MR, Maynadie M, et al. Agranular CD4+ CD56+ hematodermic neoplasm' (blastic NK-cell lymphoma) originates from a population of CD56+ precursor cells related to plasmacytoid monocytes. Am J Surg Pathol 2002;26(7): 852–62.
4. Pagano L, Valentini CG, Pulsoni A, et al. Blastic plasmacytoid dendritic cell neoplasm with leukemic presentation: an Italian multicenter study. Haematologica 2013;98(2):239–46.
5. Pagano L, Valentini CG, Grammatico S, et al. Blastic plasmacytoid dendritic cell neoplasm: diagnostic criteria and therapeutical approaches. Br J Haematol 2016; 174(2):188–202.
6. Pemmaraju N, Lane AA, Sweet KL, et al. Tagraxofusp in blastic plasmacytoid dendritic-cell neoplasm. N Engl J Med 2019;380(17):1628–37.
7. Kharfan-Dabaja MA, Lazarus HM, Nishihori T, et al. Diagnostic and therapeutic advances in blastic plasmacytoid dendritic cell neoplasm: a focus on hematopoietic cell transplantation. Biol Blood Marrow Transplant 2013;19(7):1006–12.
8. Roos-Weil D, Dietrich S, Boumendil A, et al. Stem cell transplantation can provide durable disease control in blastic plasmacytoid dendritic cell neoplasm: a retrospective study from the European Group for Blood and Marrow Transplantation. Blood 2013;121(3):440–6.
9. Aoki T, Suzuki R, Kuwatsuka Y, et al. Long-term survival following autologous and allogeneic stem cell transplantation for blastic plasmacytoid dendritic cell neoplasm. Blood 2015;125(23):3559–62.

10. Kharfan-Dabaja MA, Al Malki MM, Deotare U, et al. Haematopoietic cell transplantation for blastic plasmacytoid dendritic cell neoplasm: a North American multicentre collaborative study. Br J Haematol 2017;179(5):781–9.

11. Leclerc M, Peffault de Latour R, Michallet M, et al. Can a reduced-intensity conditioning regimen cure blastic plasmacytoid dendritic cell neoplasm? Blood 2017;129(9):1227–30.

12. Gooley TA, Chien JW, Pergam SA, et al. Reduced mortality after allogeneic hematopoietic-cell transplantation. N Engl J Med 2010;363(22):2091–101.

13. Hsieh MM, Kang EM, Fitzhugh CD, et al. Allogeneic hematopoietic stem-cell transplantation for sickle cell disease. N Engl J Med 2009;361(24):2309–17.

14. Kolb HJ, Schattenberg A, Goldman JM, et al. Graft-versus-leukemia effect of donor lymphocyte transfusions in marrow grafted patients. Blood 1995;86(5): 2041–50.

15. Kharfan-Dabaja MA, Labopin M, Polge E, et al. Association of second allogeneic hematopoietic cell transplant vs donor lymphocyte infusion with overall survival in patients with acute myeloid leukemia relapse. JAMA Oncol 2018;4(9):1245–53.

16. El-Jurdi N, Reljic T, Kumar A, et al. Efficacy of adoptive immunotherapy with donor lymphocyte infusion in relapsed lymphoid malignancies. Immunotherapy 2013; 5(5):457–66.

17. Dalle S, Beylot-Barry M, Bagot M, et al. Blastic plasmacytoid dendritic cell neoplasm: is transplantation the treatment of choice? Br J Dermatol 2010; 162(1):74–9.

18. Kharfan-Dabaja MA, Reljic T, Murthy HS, et al. Allogeneic hematopoietic cell transplantation is an effective treatment for blastic plasmacytoid dendritic cell neoplasm in first complete remission: systematic review and meta-analysis. Clin Lymphoma Myeloma Leuk 2018;18(11):703–9.e1.

19. Reimer P, Rudiger T, Kraemer D, et al. What is CD4+CD56+ malignancy and how should it be treated? Bone Marrow Transplant 2003;32(7):637–46.

20. Neelapu SS, Locke FL, Bartlett NL, et al. Axicabtagene ciloleucel CAR T-cell therapy in refractory large B-cell lymphoma. N Engl J Med 2017;377(26):2531–44.

21. Schuster SJ, Bishop MR, Tam CS, et al. Tisagenlecleucel in adult relapsed or refractory diffuse large B-cell lymphoma. N Engl J Med 2019;380(1):45–56.

22. Maude SL, Laetsch TW, Buechner J, et al. Tisagenlecleucel in children and young adults with B-cell lymphoblastic leukemia. N Engl J Med 2018;378(5):439–48.

23. Olweus J, BitMansour A, Warnke R, et al. Dendritic cell ontogeny: a human dendritic cell lineage of myeloid origin. Proc Natl Acad Sci U S A 1997;94(23): 12551–6.

24. MacDonald KP, Munster DJ, Clark GJ, et al. Characterization of human blood dendritic cell subsets. Blood 2002;100(13):4512–20.

25. Mardiros A, Dos Santos C, McDonald T, et al. T cells expressing CD123-specific chimeric antigen receptors exhibit specific cytolytic effector functions and anti-tumor effects against human acute myeloid leukemia. Blood 2013;122(18): 3138–48.

26. Guzman ML, Sugita M, Zong H, et al. Allogeneic Tcrα/β deficient CAR T-cells targeting CD123 prolong overall survival of AML patient-derived xenografts. Blood 2016;128(22):765.

27. Dohner H, Estey E, Grimwade D, et al. Diagnosis and management of AML in adults: 2017 ELN recommendations from an international expert panel. Blood 2017;129(4):424–47.

28. Al-Hussaini M, Rettig MP, Ritchey JK, et al. Targeting CD123 in acute myeloid leukemia using a T-cell-directed dual-affinity retargeting platform. Blood 2016; 127(1):122–31.

29. Montero J, Stephansky J, Cai T, et al. Blastic plasmacytoid dendritic cell neoplasm is dependent on BCL2 and sensitive to venetoclax. Cancer Discov 2017;7(2):156–64.

30. DiNardo CD, Rausch CR, Benton C, et al. Clinical experience with the BCL2-inhibitor venetoclax in combination therapy for relapsed and refractory acute myeloid leukemia and related myeloid malignancies. Am J Hematol 2018;93(3): 401–7.

Moving?

Make sure your subscription moves with you!

To notify us of your new address, find your **Clinics Account Number** (located on your mailing label above your name), and contact customer service at:

Email: journalscustomerservice-usa@elsevier.com

800-654-2452 (subscribers in the U.S. & Canada)
314-447-8871 (subscribers outside of the U.S. & Canada)

Fax number: 314-447-8029

Elsevier Health Sciences Division
Subscription Customer Service
3251 Riverport Lane
Maryland Heights, MO 63043

*To ensure uninterrupted delivery of your subscription, please notify us at least 4 weeks in advance of move.